FAROOK AL-AZZAWI

MBChB, MA (Cantab.), PhD, FRCOG

Senior Lecturer
Honorary Consultant in Obstetrics and Gynaecology
University of Leicester School of Medicine
Leicester Royal Infirmary
UK

childbirth and obstetric techniques

SECOND EDITION

Mosby

London • Philadelphia • St Louis • Sydney • Tokyo

Project Manager:	Dave Burin
Development Editor:	Gina Almond
Designer:	Paul Phillips
Layout Artist:	Rob Curran
Cover Designer:	Paul Phillips
Illustrator:	Lynda Payne
Production Controller:	Hamish Adamson
Indexer:	Laurence Errington
Publisher:	Richard Furn

First edition published in 1990 by Wolfe Publishing Ltd

This edition published in 1998 by Mosby, an imprint of Mosby International Limited
Copyright © 1998 Mosby International Limited
Printed in Barcelona, Spain, by Grafos S.A. Arte sobre papel
ISBN 0 7234 3099 3

For full details of all Mosby titles, please write to Mosby International Limited, Lynton House, 7–12 Tavistock Square, London WC1H 9LB, UK.

A CIP catalogue record for this book is available from the British Library.

Library of Congress Cataloging-in-Publication Data applied for.

Contents

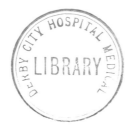

Preface to 2nd Edition

The continuing demands for an illustrated step-by-step book on childbirth and obstetric manoeuvres have encouraged me to work on this second edition of the Atlas. In it, I have endeavoured to update concepts pertinent to present-day antenatal care, ultrasound scanning and intrapartum care. A number of pictures have been updated, diagrams have been upgraded and a few new picture are added.

The progressive move to devolve intrapartum care to midwifery personnel inevitably results in dilution of the experience gained by medical students and junior trainees in the management of normal labour, and consequently lessens their ability to perform assisted deliveries, be they vaginal or abdominal. This book will serve as a pictorial reference through which the intended readership may understand the steps involved in any particular technique.

The sections on 'Pain Relief in Labour' and 'Resuscitation of the Newborn' have been rewritten, and I would like to record my thanks to the contributors for their continued support.

I felt it necessary to add a section on the emergency management of postpartum shock resulting from postpartum haemorrhage, uterine rupture and acute inversion of the uterus, and have emphasized the initial resuscitative steps required pending the arrival of a more senior colleague. This addition may serve as a reminder that the complete normality and safety of childbirth may be considered only in retrospect, at least in medical terms.

My thanks to the readership of the first edition, whose comments and remarks have resulted in this work.

Acknowledgements

The section on resuscitation of the newborn was written by Dr Paul Ward, Senior Registrar in Paediatrics, Addenbrooke's Hospital, Cambridge; and the section on obstetric anaesthesia and analgesia was contributed by Dr Saffana Shawket, Anaesthetist and Research Fellow in Clinical Pharmacology, Cambridge University. My teacher, Mr J.F. Pearson, Reader in Obstetrics and Gynaecology, University Hospital of Wales, Cardiff, has kindly agreed to publish his technique of 'en caule' caesarean section for the delivery of the premature baby in this book.

I would like to acknowledge the help of my patients, without whom this work could not have been completed. The help of the midwives and theatre staff has been tremendous and they accommodated the extra procedures with enthusiasm. Mr Allan Davidson, Medical Photographer, Norfolk and Norwich Hospital, has been remarkable with his keenness and patience; the majority of the photographs were taken by him, often after midnight! The staff of the ultrasound scanning unit at the Rosie Maternity Hospital, Cambridge, have been very helpful in gathering suitable cases for presentation; in particular I would like to thank Mrs Sylvia Bishop, Mrs Margaret Johnson and Mrs Stephanie Williams.

My colleagues have been very generous in reading and criticizing the text, and in offering their time to collect these cases, in particular Dr Catherine Bangham, Mr R.W. Stone and Dr Wen Lim; and a special thank you to Dr Christine Robinson of St Thomas's Hospital, London.

Finally, I record my great appreciation for the excellent updated line artwork in this edition. These renditions, prepared by Lynda Payne, in many instances evolved from the skilful and painstakingly drawn illustrations prepared for the 1st edition by Rosie Watts.

Preface to 1st Edition

When I began to work on this Atlas, I remembered the days of my undergraduate training in obstetrics. The mechanics described in the textbooks did not correspond to my imagined steps of childbirth. As the clinical sessions passed by, I found that I had not seen a breech, twins, or even a Kjelland's forceps delivery performed. Many precious hours were spent trying to imagine the clinical situation and relate it to the acquired experience. It was even more demanding when I started postgraduate training. The criteria followed and the decisions made by my senior colleagues appeared rather mystifying, especially during the first two months, and I had to refer to a number of textbooks in an attempt to appreciate their instructions. I was not alone in that game.

The feedback I have received through my teaching of the mechanics of labour and delivery and the techniques of operative obstetrics showed that almost all the students understood the textbook better after they were shown a series of pictures depicting the sequence of events in a particular labour. This was applicable across the board: student midwives, medical students and even senior house officers.

Moreover, obstetric teaching in practice has always been hampered by the special need of the parturient for privacy. The situation is usually discussed in whispers, lest the mother, or even the father for that matter, becomes confused and terrified by the jargon.

Throughout the Atlas, I try to keep the presentation as pragmatic as possible, to emphasize the practical aspects of obstetric techniques and to relate directly to the daily experience on labour wards. I must stress at this juncture that my efforts in this book are not meant to replace any textbooks, but rather to complement their teachings.

The recent developments in obstetrics have gradually transformed the subject into a clinical science rather than a pure art, for example, screening against congenital anomalies and growth problems, as well as the provision of intensive medical care to manage maternal diseases that complicate pregnancy. In the first part of the book, I therefore briefly touch upon the policies and techniques that helped to accomplish optimal present-day antenatal care.

In the second, third and fourth parts of the book, I describe the mechanics of normal labour and, in particular, the mechanics of the second stage, together with possible complications that may arise in the course of an apparently normal labour. Even in the case of uneventful antenatal care, normal labour may become complicated by abnormally slow progress, a poor fetal heart rate pattern and fetal metabolic acidosis. There may be mechanical difficulties with the delivery, as in shoulder dystocia, a baby that is slow to breathe, failure to procure the placenta, and the need to repair the episiotomy. Owing to the fact that in many instances these events appear with dramatic speed, I believe that any person in charge of a particular delivery must be able to act rapidly to deal with these emergencies, if immediate help is not available.

The fifth part of the book deals with operative vaginal delivery, and includes vacuum extraction, forceps delivery and rotational manoeuvres to effect the delivery of the head. At the beginning of this fifth section, I stress the importance of decision-making processes and the limits beyond which a junior trainee has to seek advice, before embarking on an operative delivery.

Breech delivery and the management of twins in the second stage occupy the sixth and seventh sections of the book. These two situations demand higher technical skills than even the performance of a caesarean section, and an experienced obstetrician is obviously needed at a moment's notice when, for example, the after-coming head extends or the arm of the second twin prolapses. The final section of the book describes the caesarean section operation and its three main types.

Finally, I hope that this book will fulfil its intended role in the teaching of obstetrics, and fill the gap in the obstetric library.

Dedicated to Saffana, William and Andrew

Chapter ONE

Antenatal Care

Sociocultural changes over the past century have resulted in a steady decline in maternal and perinatal morbidity and mortality. It is therefore not surprising that, in present day practice, prematurity and abnormal fetal development are major causative factors of perinatal loss. From the moment of conception, genetic factors derived from both parents confer upon the developing fetus the necessary defences against most of the dangers that it has to face *in utero* and outside. **Figures 1.1** and **1.2** represent the spectacular start of these processes, and illustrate the enormous wealth of genetic programmes being stored in the two pronuclei (**Fig. 1.1**).

Environmental factors have profound effects on fetal development and growth, although these may be alleviated, at least partially, through a well-structured system of antenatal care.

THE SCOPE OF ANTENATAL CARE

Antenatal care is a clinical exercise designed to ensure the safe and healthy conclusion of pregnancy for both mother and baby. The majority of pregnant women are healthy and deliver, in most cases, normal healthy babies. However, risks to the mother or the baby, or both, may develop during the course of pregnancy and labour, with surprising rapidity and disastrous consequences. Obstetricians have therefore tried to formulate lists of risk factors, on the basis of which, pregnant women who fulfil one or more of the stated criteria can be classified as carrying a high-risk pregnancy. When the presence of a certain risk, or risks, is identified (for example pregnancy associated with diabetes mellitus, pre-eclampsia or renal disease), the mother is enrolled in an intensive monitoring programme designed to minimize the effect of such a condition. However, the major challenge to all obstetricians still lies in the fact that there is no way to quantify any particular risk in the individual patient, hence there is a high false-positive inclusion rate in any selection exercise. By the same token, there is no test sufficiently accurate to eliminate all false-negative cases.

Adverse nutritional and other environmental factors are no longer common features of present-day antenatal care

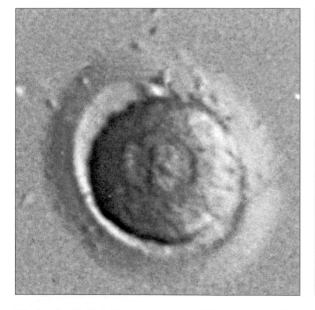

Fig. 1.1 Fertilization of a human oocyte and the appearance of pronuclei.

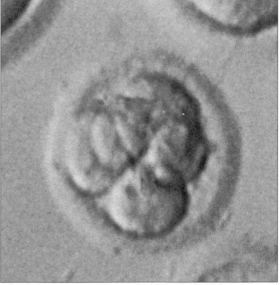

Fig. 1.2 Human embryo (four-cell stage).

in the Western world, but other problems do exist: morphological variation of the pelvis (e.g. after fractures involving the pelvic bones) may alter its capacity and result in difficulties analogous to those caused by rickets; anaemia still occurs, causing maternal fatigue, a possible reduction in the mother's ability to cope with any postpartum blood loss and even fetal growth retardation. Smoking, alcoholism, drug abuse and sexually transmitted diseases are significant causes of perinatal morbidity and mortality, and of future physical, mental and social handicap. These adverse sociological and economic factors may be alleviated through health education, provided in antenatal clinics and through associated activities such as parentcraft classes. Such efforts are reinforced by those of community midwives, district nurses and health visitors.

Pre-eclampsia remains as enigmatic a disorder as it was 50 years ago; its treatment and prevention remain major concerns in the antenatal care of today.

In some cases, a special level of expertise in antenatal care is required: for example, pregnancies in mothers with insulin-dependent diabetes, or pregnancies in mothers who have successfully undergone corrective surgery of major heart defects or have received an organ transplant. Owing to vast improvements in medical and surgical management, most such patients do now survive long enough to be able to reproduce and to look after their progeny, even though the physiological burden of pregnancy may complicate their otherwise stabilized conditions.

Methods allowing antenatal diagnosis of fetal malformations, chromosomal abnormalities and an ever-expanding list of metabolic disorders have quite recently been introduced into routine clinical obstetric practice. Antenatal diagnosis relies, in the main, on morphometric features of the growing conceptus, assessed by ultrasound scanning, which is backed up by amniocentesis, chorion villus sampling and cordocentesis. These techniques enable the application of various biochemical and molecular biological procedures to cells grown *in vitro*. The scope of antenatal care is thus wide and, if a high success rate is to be achieved, requires special experience in a number of situations, perhaps even including fetal therapy. Today, the field is being staffed jointly by the obstetrician, the clinical geneticist and the biochemist.

ULTRASOUND SCANNING

Ultrasound scanning represents an integral part of present-day antenatal care in the Western world and in many of the developing countries. It has transformed antenatal care from being largely a matter of guesswork as to the gestational age, to the ability to provide accurate dating of a pregnancy to within 7 days and to document fetal growth, particularly when fetal growth retardation is suspected. The main measurements used to monitor growth are the biparietal diameter, abdominal circumference, head circumference : abdominal circumference ratio and length of femur. In addition, ultrasound scanning is an essential tool in the diagnosis of fetal abnormalities, especially those shown in **Figures 1.3a–1.13b**.

Ultrasound scanning has also simplified the diagnosis of multiple pregnancy early in gestation (**Figs 1.14 & 1.15**).

The development of complications early in pregnancy can also be identified with the aid of ultrasound scanning (**Figs 1.16a–1.25b**).

MAGNETIC RESONANCE IMAGING

Technical advances in obstetric imaging have introduced magnetic resonance imaging (MRI), which is currently being evaluated in some research centres. MRI is based on the principle that atoms aligned within a strong magnetic

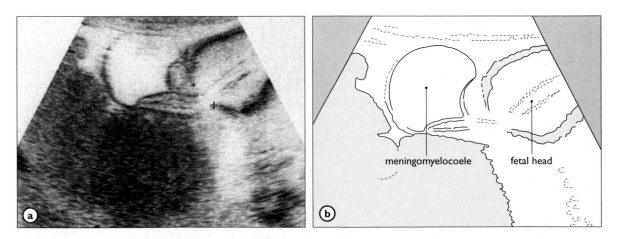

Fig. 1.3a & b Meningomyelocoele.

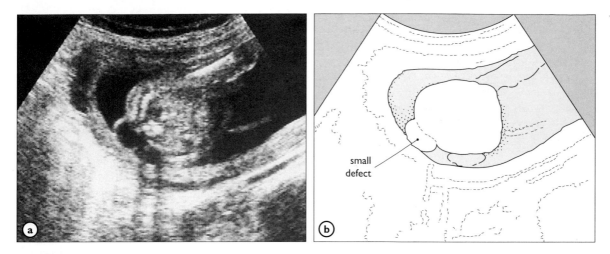

Fig. 1.4a & b Spina bifida: small defect. (**Fig.1.4a** *courtesy of Dr K Krarup.*)

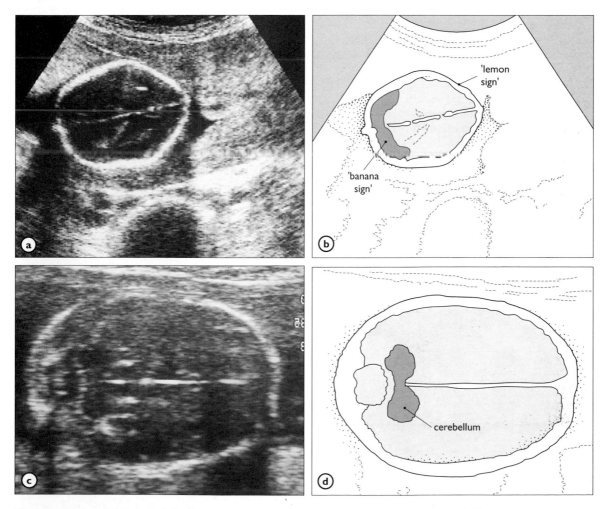

Fig. 1.5a–d Spina bifida: 'banana sign' **a & b**, in which the outline of the cerebellum looks like a banana, probably because of the herniation at the spinal defect – the outline of the skull resembles a lemon ('lemon sign'); **c & d** portray the outline of a normal skull and normal cerebellum.

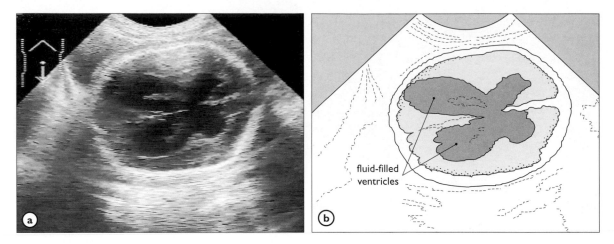

Fig. 1.6a & b Hydrocephalus: the brain is being replaced by dilated cerebral ventricles.

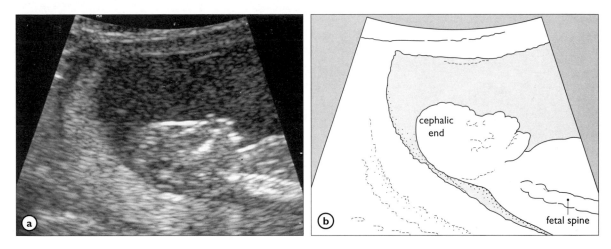

Fig. 1.7a & b Anencephaly: failure of development of the cerebral vesicles.

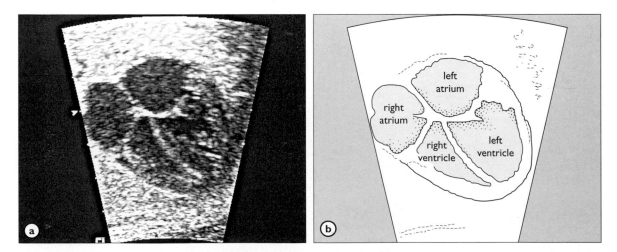

Fig. 1.8a & b Normal appearance of four-chamber view of the fetal heart – usually excludes the presence of a major congenital heart defect. (**Fig. 1.8a** *courtesy of Dr J Konje.*)

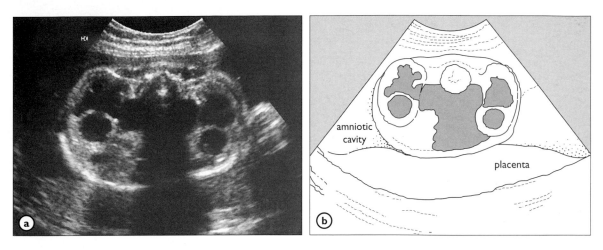

Fig. 1.9a & b Congenital defect of the kidneys: renal cyst of the left kidney. The inability to visualize the urinary bladder should alert the observer to the possibility of renal agenesis. Oligohydramnios is manifest. (**Fig.1.9a** *courtesy of Dr J Konje*.)

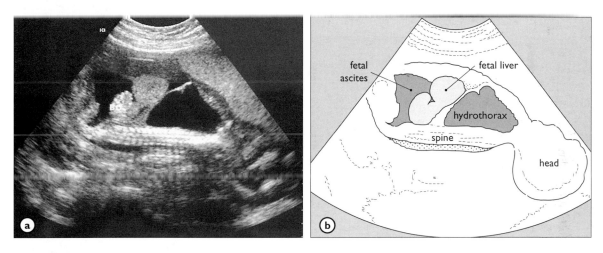

Fig. 1.10a & b Development of ascites and hydrops: this condition may be idiopathic, or may develop as a result of isoimmunization or intrauterine fetal infection. (**Fig.1.10a** *courtesy of Dr J Konje*.)

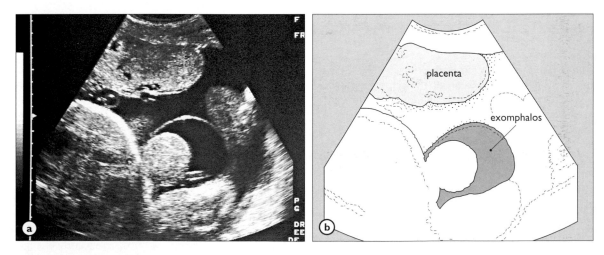

Fig. 1.11a & b Defects of the anterior abdominal wall: exomphalos. Exomphalos is the herniation of abdominal contents, intestines and sometimes also the liver. There is a covering sac that consists of amnion and peritoneum. This condition is associated with a high incidence of chromosomal abnormalities. (**Fig.1.11a** *courtesy of Dr J Konje*.)

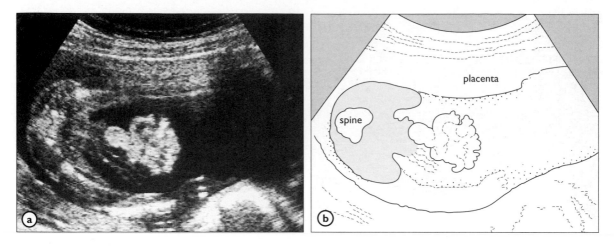

Fig. 1.12a & b Gastroschisis: intestinal herniation through a defect in the anterior abdominal wall. In contrast to exomphalos, there is no sac and the intestines are covered with an inflammatory exudate. (**Fig.1.12a** *courtesy of Dr J Konje.*)

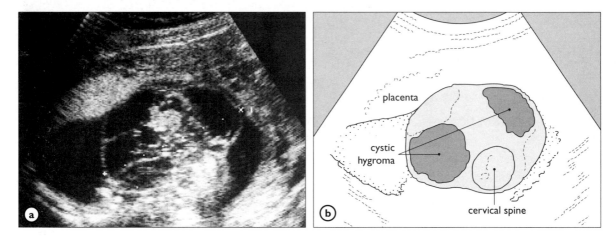

Fig. 1.13a & b Turner's syndrome was diagnosed (and confirmed cytogenetically) in this patient when a cystic hygroma was noted. (**Fig.1.13a** *courtesy of Dr J Konje.*)

field respond to certain radiofrequency waves by re-emitting some of the absorbed energy. The technique is of limited value in imaging the upper abdomen, because of the effect of ventilatory movements. Similarly, its efficiency in screening the fetus during the first and second trimesters is reduced because of fetal movement, but developments are under way that aim to shorten the time of exposure and reduce the angle of deflection, and thus to obtain structural details of the fetus.

However, MRI can be used to produce excellent images of the female pelvis in the third trimester of pregnancy, and is invaluable for studying the details of the pelvis, where there is only a limited effect of ventilatory movements. The technique has the distinct advantage of being safe, as it does not utilize any form of ionizing radiation.

It is expected that this technology will introduce the ability to conduct biochemical and physiological evaluation of fetal tissue *in utero* and thus become a powerful non-invasive investigative tool (**Fig. 1.26**).

AMNIOCENTESIS

Amniocentesis (**Figs 1.27–1.29**) is the sampling of amniotic fluid, for antenatal diagnosis of chromosomal and biochemical abnormalities by means of the examination of shed fetal cells and the amniotic fluid itself. It is usually performed after 16 weeks' gestation, so that the loss of the aspirated fluid will not significantly change the volume of the uterine cavity, resulting in uterine contractions. Performance of amniocentesis in the second

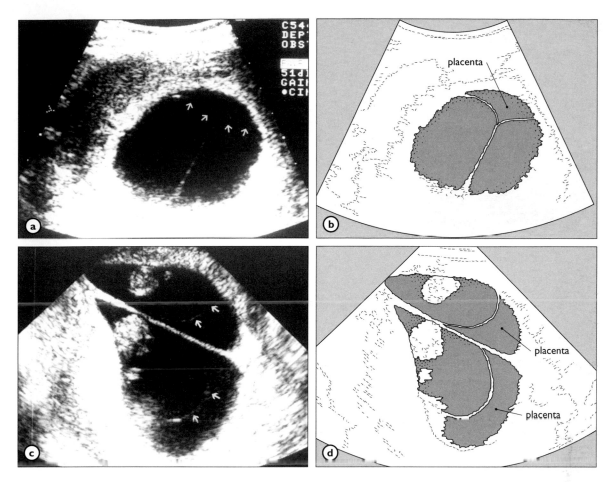

Fig. 1.14a–d Twins: two sacs and two fetal poles. The amnion and chorion are shown in this early stage of pregnancy. The silhouette of the fetal membrane configuration may help to identifiy chorionicity of the placenta. A T-sign indicates a monochorionic placenta (**a & b**), which is associated with increased fetal morbidity and mortality. A dichorionic placenta is demonstrated with the λ-sign in **c & d**.

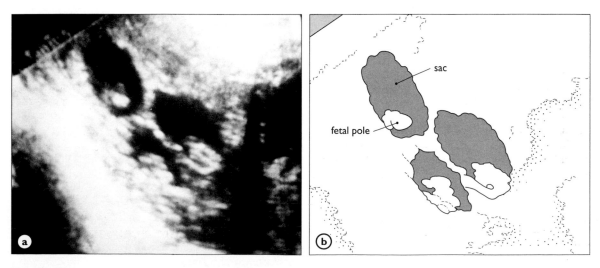

Fig. 1.15a & b Triplets: three sacs and three fetal poles.

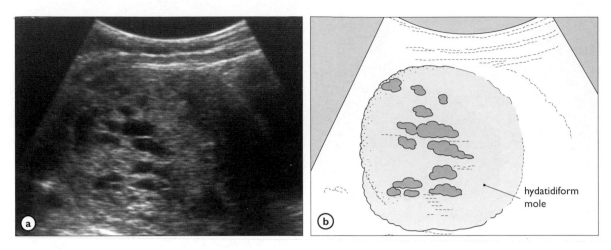

Fig. 1.16a & b Hydatidiform mole: note the cotton-wool appearance with cystic spaces – a characteristic sonographic feature of trophoblastic disease.

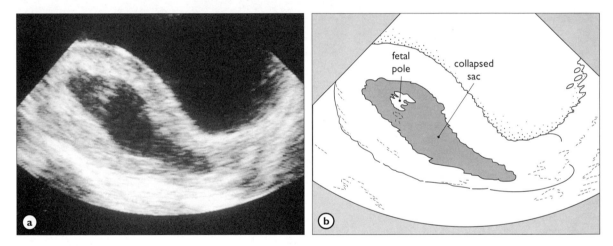

Fig. 1.17a & b Missed abortion: the collapsed sac is smaller than the size expected for the gestational age; the fetal pole is present, but the fetal heart movement was not detected.

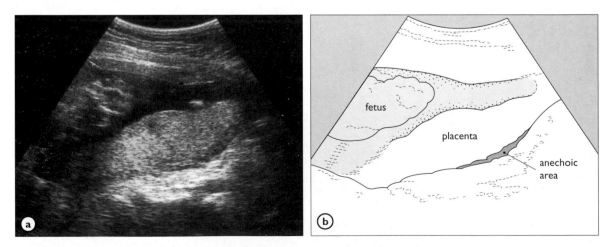

Fig. 1.18a & b Ultrasonic placentography, or placental localization, has significantly contributed to the care of patients who present with antepartum haemorrhage. Shown here is a case of a low-lying placenta complicated by placental abruption; note the anechoeic area between the placenta and the uterine wall.

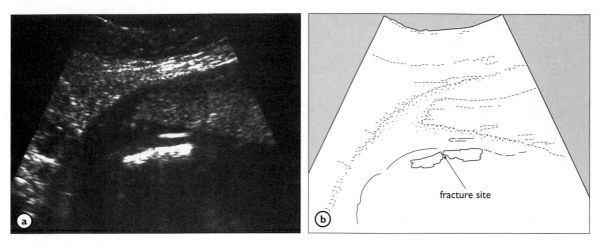

Fig. 1.19a & b Osteogenesis imperfecta is a syndrome of brittle bones characterized by a high propensity for fractures. It is associated with fetal growth retardation. (**Fig.1.19a** *courtesy of Dr K Krarup.*)

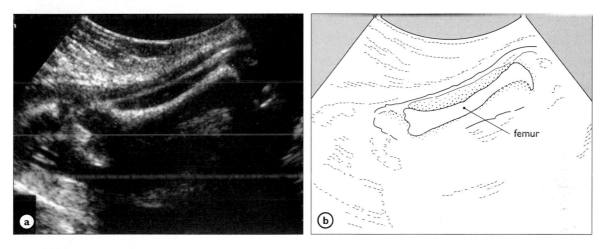

Fig. 1.20a & b Measurement of the length of the femur by means of ultrasound is a useful parameter for monitoring linear growth of the fetus. (**Fig.1.20a** *courtesy of Dr J Konje.*)

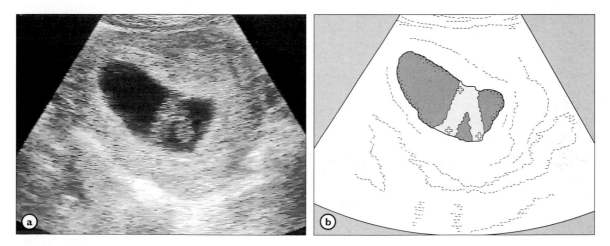

Fig. 1.21a & b Conjoined twins can be diagnosed in early pregnancy. The two fetuses move together and are fixed at one region. In this case, two fetal hearts have been identified.

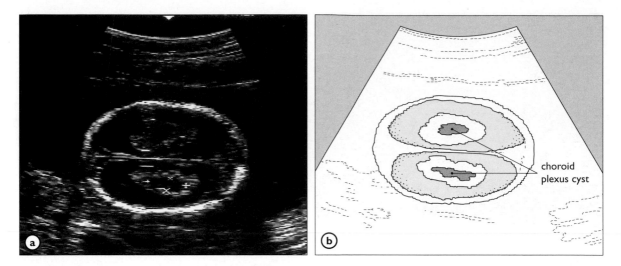

Fig. 1.22a & b Choroid plexus cyst: a cystic abnormality of the choroid plexus overlying the cerebral ventricle. It may be transient and shrinks or disappears at 22–26 weeks' gestation. There is a relatively high association with trisomy 18, in which other morphological features of the syndrome, such as club foot, can be identified.

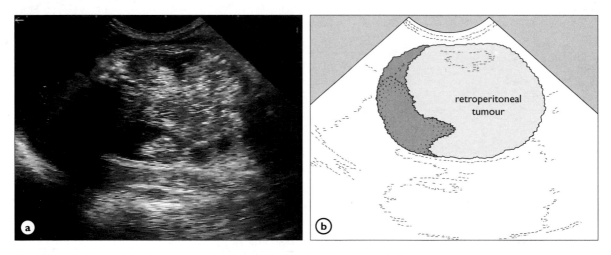

Fig. 1.23a & b Retroperitoneal tumours may be diagnosed *in utero*. In this case, the pathology was a retroperitoneal teratoma and there may be an associated fetal hydrops.

trimester lessens the chance of traumatizing the fetus, owing to the abundance of liquor present at that stage. However, investigators are trying to evaluate the advantages of such a procedure performed earlier in pregnancy, for example after 12 weeks' gestation. Larger studies are awaited to examine the merits and comparative safety of such a practice.

CHORION VILLUS SAMPLING

In an attempt to obtain tissue of fetal origin at an earlier stage of pregnancy than that at which amniocentesis is performed (16 weeks' gestation), chorion villus sampling (CVS) has been developed. This technique allows the culture of actively dividing cells, as opposed to the shed cells

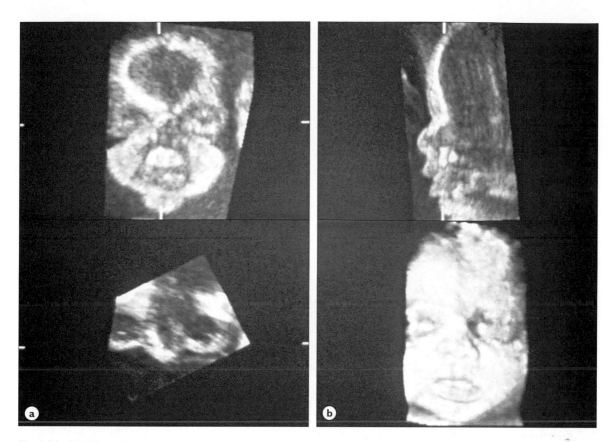

Fig. 1.24a & b Three-dimensional ultrasound scanning has introduced a significant degree of precision by adding a spacial impression into the field of fetal imaging. Congenital malformation may be more clearly identified. (*Courtesy of Kretztechnik AG, Zipf, Austria.*)

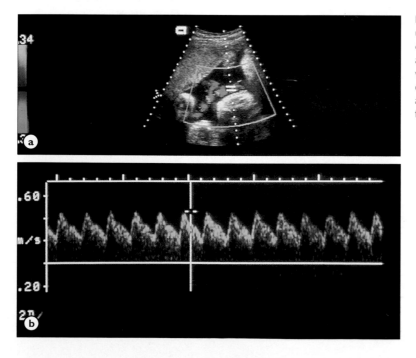

Fig. 1.25a & b Doppler imaging of umbilical blood flow: **a**, colour Doppler image of the umbilical cord, revealing the coiling appearance of the cord. The flow in the vessels is depicted in blue and red, depending on its direction; **b**, power Doppler image of an umbilical artery, showing a normal blood flow velocity with EDF.

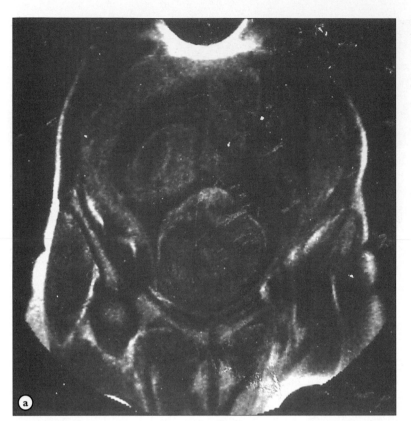

Fig. 1.26a & b MRI: coronal section of the lower abdomen of a pregnant woman, showing the contents of the uterus. The head and fetal parts are clearly delineated. (**Fig. 1.26a** *courtesy of Professor M Symonds, Nottingham.*)

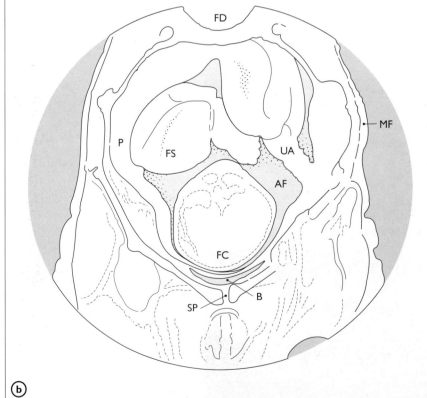

FD = field defect
MF = maternal subcutaneous fat
P   = placenta
UA = upper arm
FS = fetal shoulder
AF = amniotic fluid
FC = fetal cerebrum
B   = maternal bladder
SP = symphysis pubis

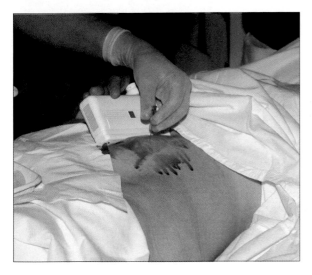

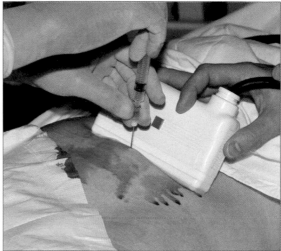

Fig. 1.27 Amniocentesis: after local infiltration of the skin with 2 ml of 1% lignocaine solution, and under sterile conditions, a 10-cm 20–22G spinal needle is introduced through the abdominal wall into the amniotic cavity, under ultrasound guidance.

Fig. 1.28 Amniocentesis: as the needle stylet is removed, clear amniotic fluid slowly wells out and can be aspirated with a syringe. Should the fluid be blood-stained, 1–2 ml is aspirated and discarded, and another syringe is attached to aspirate clear fluid.

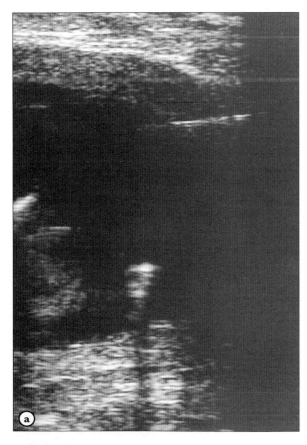

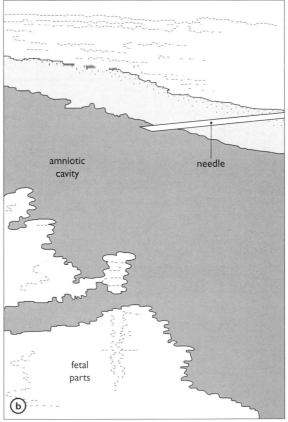

Fig. 1.29a & b Amniocentesis: the needle is in the amniotic cavity, guided by ultrasound scan, which helps it to avoid the placenta and the fetal parts.

recovered at amniocentesis, and, if an abnormality is discovered, permits termination of pregnancy at a relatively early stage. However, CVS carries a 2–3% procedure-related risk of fetal loss, which is greater than that incurred by amniocentesis.

The growth potential of chorionic villi facilitates relatively quick karyotyping, within 3–4 days. The possibility of obtaining a large cell population (greater in CVS than in amniocentesis) improves the chance that biochemical techniques may detect inborn errors of metabolism and serious inherited disorders.

Initial attempts at CVS were made via the transcervical route. However, the high rate of complications and the relative difficulty of positioning have since opened the way for the transabdominal technique: instead of being directed at the amniotic fluid pool, the 19–20G needle is aimed at the placenta, and guided by real-time ultrasound scan (**Fig. 1.30**). The operation is thus essentially similar to amniocentesis.

Other risks of CVS, if it is performed earlier than 10 weeks' gestation, include an association with a greater incidence of limb defects, but the exact mechanism for this is not known. Another problem in interpreting the results of cultured chorionic villi is the high incidence of mosaicism, which may be misinterpreted as a fetal karyotype abnormality. Confirmation by amniocentesis is required. Hence, many obstetricians are moving towards early amniocentesis, at 12–14 weeks, if karyotyping the fetus is the only test required.

FETOSCOPY

This technique (**Fig. 1.31**) has been used in the diagnosis of small fetal malformations, such as facial cleft or digital defects in families at risk from specific genetic syndromes, and for visual guidance for fetal blood sampling and skin and liver biopsy.

CORDOCENTESIS

This technique (**Fig. 1.32**) has now superseded fetoscopy for fetal blood sampling and fetal blood transfusions. In addition to being used for the prenatal diagnosis of hereditary blood disorders such as haemophilia, cordocentesis is used in the diagnosis of fetal infections such as rubella, the assessment of oxygenation and metabolism in intrauterine growth retardation and the assessment and treatment of fetal anaemia in red cell isoimmunization. It is an outpatient technique performed under local anaesthesia, and the procedure-related fetal loss is less than 1% (Nicolaides & Soothill, 1989).

ASSESSMENT OF RISKS IN THE PREGNANT WOMAN

A thorough assessment of the risks faced by the expectant mother forms the core of obstetric management. Certain factors in the patient's medical history or in her previous obstetric performance may place her in a high-risk category. Most of these risk factors have been identified in previous studies, particularly in *The Perinatal Mortality Survey* conducted in Britain in 1970, on which several of the hypotheses governing current practice are based. Pre-pregnancy counselling, particularly for women with insulin-dependent diabetes mellitus, may facilitate more efficient planning of antenatal care. A more extensive consideration of the issue of pre-pregnancy counselling is beyond the scope of this book.

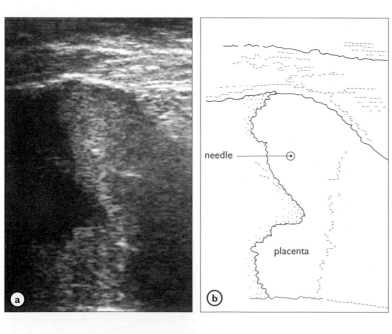

Fig. 1.30a & b CVS: the needle, seen here in cross-section, is guided by ultrasound imaging to the placenta.

needle

placenta

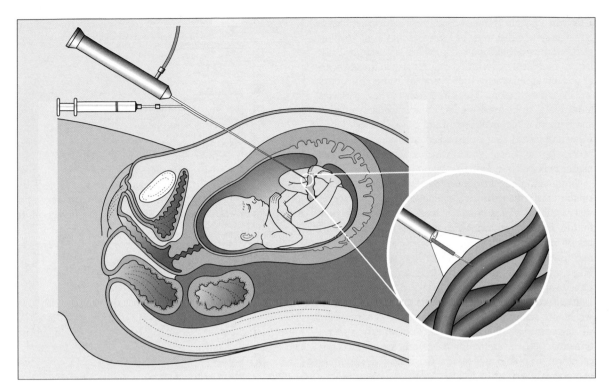

Fig. 1.31 In fetoscopy, a 1.7-mm diameter endoscope is passed transabdominally into the amniotic cavity. The endoscope is housed in a 2.2 × 2.7-mm diameter oval cannula, which has a side-channel for the introduction of needles or biopsy forceps.

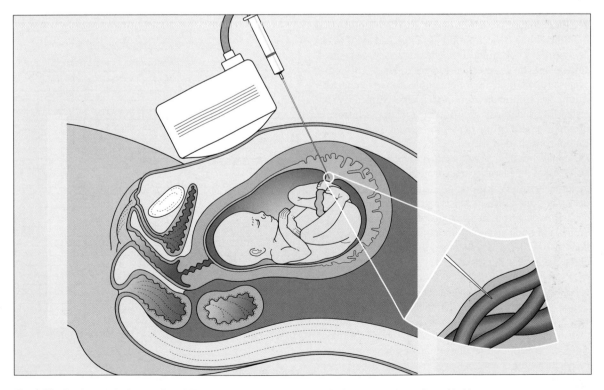

Fig. 1.32 Cordocentesis: the needle (20G) is advanced to the umbilical vein for fetal blood sampling, guided by real-time ultrasound scanning.

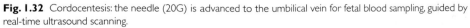

When a patient is interviewed, there is no recommended single system that must be followed, but the information gathered must be sufficiently comprehensive to cover all risk factors, and must be recorded early enough in the pregnancy to allow arrangements to be made for the necessary tests and management plans. To ensure that all the relevant aspects are satisfactorily covered, a suitable format for data gathering and retrieval is required. Boddy and co-workers developed a practical record card for use in antenatal care, which can be kept by the patient, and in which significant risk factors may be indicated by ticks in the appropriate boxes (**Fig. 1.33**).

Automation has introduced databases designed along similar lines, but with the advantages of easy storage of vast numbers of records and access at the touch of a button. Entries into the respective fields in the databases can be input via keyboard, or bar codes and light pen, and may then be used by medical, midwifery and clerical staff. These are essential tools for modern clinical practice and provide an invaluable point of reference for audit.

During the patient's first clinic visit, her weight, height and blood pressure, together with the results of urine analysis, are recorded. A general physical examination and a bimanual pelvic examination are conducted, and a cervical smear for cytology is obtained if indicated. A sample of blood is taken, and a record made of the haemoglobin concentration and cellular blood count, which should be repeated later on in pregnancy, at 28 and 36 weeks. The ABO blood group is checked, along with the rhesus status and the presence of any irregular blood group antibodies, which are checked again at 28 and 36 weeks. In rhesus-negative women, evidence of anti-rhesus antibodies, or their increasing concentration, is re-checked at 20 weeks and every 4 weeks thereafter. The presence of hepatitis B surface antigen is screened for, and titres of antibodies against rubella and treponemal infections are checked. Antibodies to human immunodeficiency virus (HIV) are tested for in high-risk groups, when there is a history of drug abuse and in women with bisexual partners, after careful consultation with the patient.

Alphafetoprotein (AFP), a protein produced by the fetal liver, crosses the placenta to the maternal circulation. A high maternal serum concentration may indicate neural tube defects and anencephaly. AFP is also increased in numerous conditions ranging from threatened abortion to Turner's syndrome and renal agenesis, among others. AFP concentrations are considered to be increased if they are >2.5 multiples of the median for the gestational age concerned. At 15–18 weeks, abnormally low levels (<0.4 multiples of the median) of AFP are associated with a greater chance of Down's syndrome – a fact that is utilized in the screening programme of the Down's syndrome risk test. This takes into account measurements of concentrations of AFP, β-subunits of human chorionic gonadotrophin and serum oestriol to calculate a risk factor for the chance of Down's syndrome being present in that pregnancy; if the risk factor is high (>1 : 200) amniocentesis may be justified in a young woman, in order to establish a definitive karyotype. An ultrasound scan is

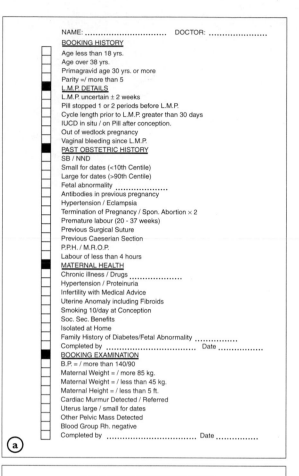

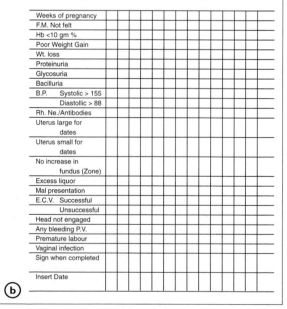

Fig. 1.33 Risk card: the front (**a**) is completed at the initial interview; on the reverse (**b**), factors arising during pregnancy are recorded. (*Courtesy of Dr K. Boddy, Edinburgh.*)

scheduled for a later date – generally at 18–19 weeks' amenorrhoea, or earlier if there is a gross discrepancy between uterine size and dates, as counted from the first day of the last menstrual period. This helps to confirm the dates and to exclude the presence of major structural abnormalities of the fetus.

OBSTETRIC PALPATION

The purpose of examining the pregnant uterus in the third trimester (**Figs 1.34–1.39**) is to ascertain the overall uterine size in relation to gestational age, to assess the fetal lie and presentation, and the descent of the presenting part into the pelvis.

When examining a pregnant uterus, it is important to remember not to leave the patient in the supine position, lest supine hypotension syndrome should develop. This occurs when the pressure of the gravid uterus compresses the inferior vena cava, impedes venous return and results in hypotension, tachycardia and fainting. The head of the examination couch must therefore be propped up, to allow the weight of the uterus to move away from the great vein.

The abdomen is exposed between the xiphisternum and the pubic region. It is important to note any surgical scar that may not have been discussed at the time when the patient's history was taken.

Engagement of the head refers to the descent of the biparietal plane of the head past the pelvic inlet. Clinically, the examiner can relate finger's breadth to the size of the fetal head and traditionally this is described in fifths. If it is estimated that only two-fifths of the head are palpable per abdomen, the head has engaged the pelvis.

In patients in whom the fetal head has already engaged the pelvis, the anterior shoulder of the fetus may be confused with the cephalic prominence. However, the manoeuvre depicted in **Figure 1.36** helps to avoid this, and may also help to assess the extent of descent of the head into the pelvis, by estimating how many fifths are palpable per abdomen. If the cephalic prominence can be felt on the same side as the small parts (arms and legs), the head is flexed and the baby is presenting by the vertex. If, however, the cephalic prominence is alongside the convexity of the back, the head is then said to be extended.

To help locate the back of the fetus, a manoeuvre described by Fairbairn in 1930 proves useful (**Figs 1.38 & 1.39**). Fairbairn's manoeuvre is particularly helpful when the obstetrician is called upon to assist in the second stage of labour, enabling the assessment of the position of the fetal head before a forceps delivery is performed, when caput succedaneum has masked the outlines of the anterior fontanelle.

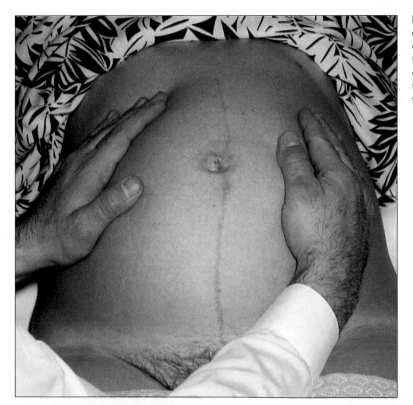

Fig. 1.34 Obstetric palpation: both of the examiner's hands are laid flat and relaxed on the abdomen to assess the contour of the uterus, the lie of the fetus and the level of the fundus. With the tips of the fingers, the examiner then assesses which part of the fetus occupies the uterine fundus.

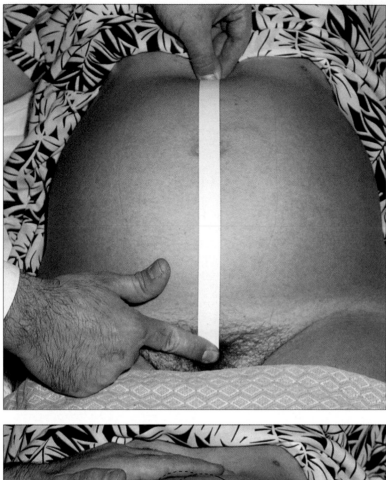

Fig. 1.35 Obstetric palpation: a tape measure, with its blank side facing upwards, is used to measure the distance between the symphysis pubis and the level of the uterine fundus. After 20 weeks' gestation, the measurement in centimetres corresponds to the duration of pregnancy in weeks, with an average variation of approximately 3 weeks, when measurements are taken after 30 weeks.

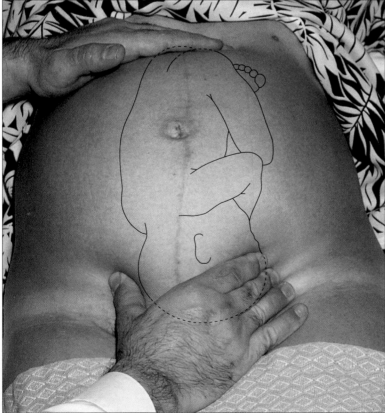

Fig. 1.36 Obstetric palpation: the fetal pole above the symphysis pubis is grasped gently but firmly with the thumb and fingers of the right hand. The contour and consistency of the fetal pole that occupies the lower part of the uterus can then be examined and compared with the other pole in the fundus.

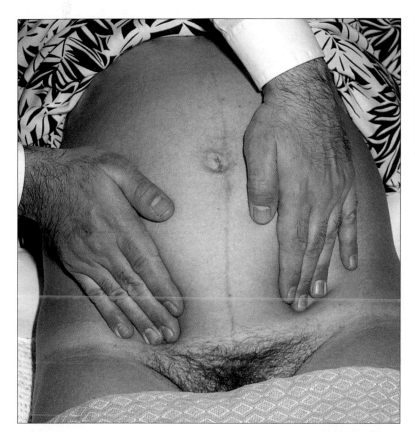

Fig. 1.37 Obstetric palpation: if the presentation is cephalic, the examiner faces the mother's feet and presses with the first three fingers of each hand on the sides of the fetal head, in the direction of the pelvic inlet. The fingers of one hand usually manage to slip in the direction of the pelvic inlet, whilst those of the other hand, being alongside the cephalic prominence, are obstructed. This manoeuvre helps to assess the degree of flexion of the fetal head.

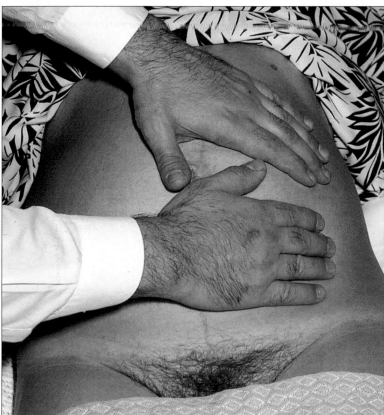

Fig. 1.38 Fairbairn's manoeuvre: initially, both hands are laid flat and relaxed on the far side of the uterus, away from the examiner.

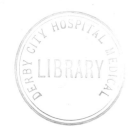

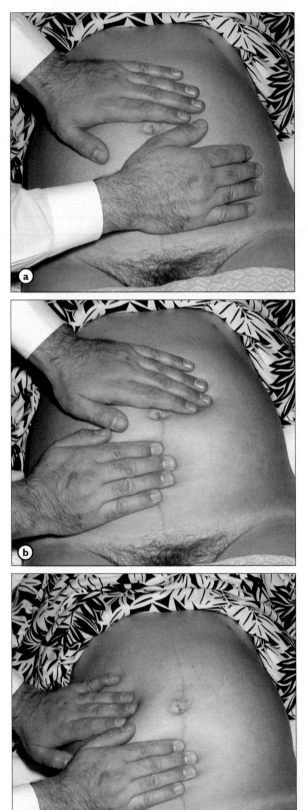

Figs. 1.39a–c Fairbairn's manoeuvre: by moving the hands backwards (towards the examiner) one hand at a time and pressing with the fingertips of the other hand, it is easy to locate the convexity of the fetal back and the concavity of the fetal front, which contains the small parts.

Chapter TWO

The Mechanism of Childbirth

Labour is a normal physiological process that commences with uterine contractions of increasing frequency, duration and pain, which permit the effacement and dilatation of the cervix such that the fetus passes through the birth canal and is safely delivered.

In order to understand the mechanics that culminate in childbirth, one may begin by considering the conventional divisions of the components of labour: powers, passages and passenger. For a normal delivery to take place, each of these three factors must fulfil its own role and interact efficiently with the other two factors.

THE POWERS: THE UTERINE MUSCLE

The increase in frequency and strength of uterine contractions appears to be a self-propagating mechanism: as a result of uterine contractions, subtle changes in the biochemical milieu and the excitability of uterine muscle fibres occur, which affects their shape; this predisposes the uterine muscle fibres to more pronounced changes after each contraction. The essential feature of uterine muscle contraction is 'retraction', whereby, at the end of each contraction, the muscle fibres retain some of the shortening achieved. The contraction wave starts at one uterine cornu and spreads down to the rest of the organ – a process referred to as 'fundal dominance'.

The bulk of the tissue that makes up the upper uterine segment is composed of smooth muscle fibres, whereas in the lower uterine segment and cervix the smooth muscle mass makes up only 10% of the tissue. Successive uterine contractions start at the uterine fundus and, as the muscles undergo retraction, result in the progressive thinning of the lower uterine segment, and effacement of the cervix. As the first stage of labour progresses, the upper segment of the uterus becomes increasingly thick and contains a greater muscle mass; a stronger pressure gradually mounts in the active upper segment, and drives the contents of the uterus into the lower segment and cervix, the smooth muscle fibres of which undergo progressive thinning. The demarcation between the upper and the lower segments of the uterus on its inner side is called the 'physiological retraction ring' (**Fig. 2.1**).

This process, which constitutes the first stage of labour, begins as early as the last few weeks of pregnancy, with the appearance of Braxton Hicks' contractions, but becomes more noticeable at the beginning of labour. These contractions eventually transform the cervix from a cylindrical organ with a narrow orifice, into an opening that

allows the passage of the fetal head into the pelvic cavity. The cervix, at the end of the first stage of labour, merges almost completely with the lower uterine segment – the state of full dilatation of the cervix.

THE PASSAGES

THE BONY PELVIS

The bony pelvis is formed by the two innominate bones (created by the fusion of three bones: the os pubis, os ischium and os ilium), which bound the pelvic cavity on each side. The innominate bones converge anteriorly to join both sides of the symphysis pubis, and are held together posteriorly by the sacrum, through the sacroiliac joints. The shape of the pelvic cavity is essentially cylindrical, but the birth canal curves forward slightly at its caudal end, at an angle of about 90° – hence its description as the 'J-' or 'L-shaped canal' when viewed in the sagittal plane (**Fig. 2.2**). The arcuate lines and the sacral promontory form the divide between the 'false' pelvis superiorly and the 'true' pelvis inferiorly. The shape of this rim is critical to

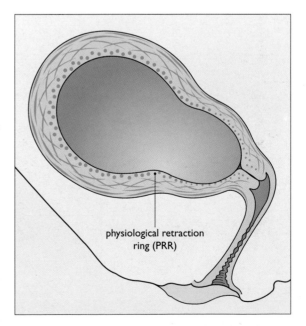

Fig. 2.1 The physiological retraction ring (PRR).

the process of engagement of the presenting part into the true pelvis, as it is the first determinant of the baby's path. The shape and dimensions of the bony pelvis are determined by a number of genetic, hormonal and environmental factors. Three main types are recognized: gynaecoid, android and anthropoid.

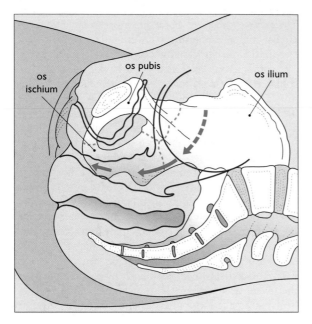

Fig. 2.2 The 'J-' or 'L-shaped' canal: a section of the pregnant pelvis in the sagittal plane; the background illustration of the bony structures helps show their relationship with the soft tissue.

The gynaecoid pelvis – the typical female pelvis (**Fig. 2.3**) – is found in about 40% of women and shows an overall rounded appearance of the cavity and a well-curved bony cage, with less prominent bony landmarks than those found on the other variants of the female pelvis, discussed below. The plane of the inlet is largely circular, with a small indentation caused by the forwardly pointing promontory of the sacrum. The body of the sacrum, produced by the fusion of the five sacral vertebrae, forms a downward curve, its concavity facing anteriorly. The curved side-walls of the pelvis are formed, from front to back, by the pubic, ischial and iliac components of the innominate bone; they are arranged such that the curvature of the sacrum is continuous with the sides of the pelvic cavity. The pelvic side-walls also contain the greater sciatic foramen, which is wide and shallow in the typical female pelvis; this feature helps the baby's head to negotiate the forwardly bent birth canal with greater ease. The plane of the pelvic outlet is rhomboid shaped, or like two triangles in different planes but joined by one side in the middle; its boundaries are the two sacrotuberous ligaments and the arch created by the pubic rami. The subpubic arch in the typical female pelvis forms a right-angle, allowing more space for the fetal head to engage the pelvic outlet, in contrast to that in the android pelvis, in which the angle is usually acute.

In the android pelvis, found in about 30–35% of women, the plane of the inlet is heavily indented by the sacral promontory, and its sides converge more acutely at the front of the pelvis, transforming the inlet into a heart-shaped plane. This encourages the baby's head to engage the pelvic inlet with the sagittal suture in either of the oblique diameters, and the occiput in the posterior position. The sacrum is rather straight and, together with the

Fig. 2.3 In a typical gynaecoid pelvis, the pelvic inlet is round, and the average diameters are as depicted.

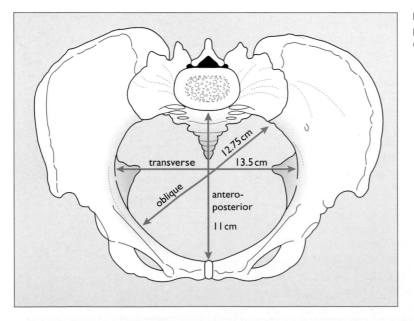

prominent ischial spines, tends to hinder the rotation of the fetal head to the occipitoanterior position.

In the anthropoid pelvis, however, which is found in about 15–20% of women, the anteroposterior diameter of the inlet is greater than its transverse diameter, giving it an oval shape. The sacrum is formed of six vertebrae, and the pelvis is generally deeper than other types. The subpubic arch is relatively narrow and the ischial spines are prominent, but the greater sciatic notch is wide. This type of pelvis favours the occipitoposterior position and, not uncommonly, the baby is born as face-to-pubis.

THE PELVIC FLOOR

The shape and structure of the pelvic floor have a major role in directing the descending fetal head through the forwardly bent lower portion of the birth canal.

On each side of the pelvic cavity, the levator ani muscle, a fan-shaped muscle, arises from the ischial spine, the white line (which overlies and is closely related to the obturator internus fascia) and the body of the pubic bone. Each comprises a pubococcygeus, iliococcygeus and a posterior ischiococcygeus (or coccygeus) muscle. The levator ani muscles from both sides converge medially, backwards and downwards, and are inserted into the coccyx and anococcygeal raphe (from the tip of the coccyx to the anorectal junction). These muscles thus form the pelvic diaphragm, which is slung around the midline body effluents.

The coccygeus muscle forms the posterior boundary of the pelvic floor, along with part of the piriformis muscle.

The pubococcygeus muscle arises from the anterior half of the white line and from the back of the body of the pubic bone; it spreads backwards and medially and above the pelvic surface of the iliococcygeus muscle to insert into the anococcygeal raphe.

The puborectalis muscle, the medial part of the pubococcygeus muscle, consists of muscle fibres that arise more anteriorly from the periosteum of the body of the pubic bone, pass backwards and at a lower level than the pubococcygeus, and form a U-shaped sling with the muscle from the other side, behind the anorectal junction, to angle it forwards. The more medial fibres form a U-shaped sling around the vagina and insert into the perineal body, forming the sphincter vaginae; the lateral walls of the lower one-third of the vagina are attached to these medial fibres. The sphincter vaginae should not be confused with the sphincter of the introitus formed by the bulbospongiosus muscle. At rest, the puborectalis muscle squeezes the rectum, vagina and urethra closed by compressing them against the pubic bone. The perineal body is the meeting point of all the superficial and deep muscles of the perineum with the levatores ani, which further enforces the architecture of the pelvic diaphragm.

This convergence of the pelvic diaphragm, as it extends from the side-walls of the pelvic cavity down to the muscular raphe in the midline, transforms the shape of the pelvic floor from a simple sheet of muscle into a gutter that contributes to the bent lower portion of the birth canal discussed above (**Fig. 2.4a&b**).

The essential role in childbirth of the gutter-shaped pelvic floor is to align the sagittal suture of the descending head with the anteroposterior diameter of the pelvic outlet. The leading part of the fetal head touches the pelvic floor and moves to the front; this is the occiput in a well-flexed head, or the sinciput in a deflexed head in the occipitoposterior position.

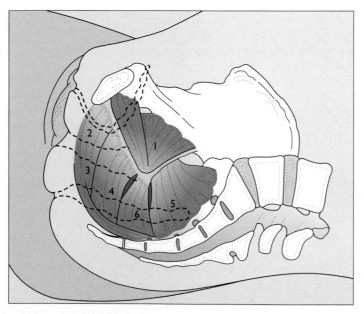

Fig. 2.4a Architecture of the pelvic diaphragm:
1 Obturator internus.
2 Puborectalis.
3 Pubococcygeus.
4 Illiococcygeus.
5 Piriformis.
6 Coccygeus.
Dotted lines illustrate relative positions of bladder, urethra, vagina and rectum

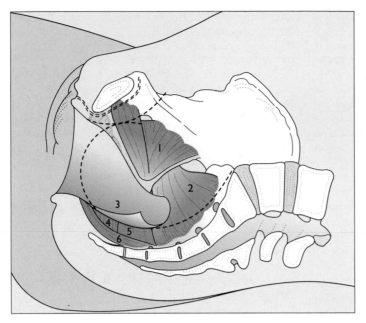

Fig. 2.4b The pelvic floor in the second stage of labour: the distended vagina is shown in the foreground to illustrate the anatomical relationship:
1. Obturator internus.
2. Piriformis.
3. Vagina
4. Iliococcygeus
5. Coccygeus.
6. Pubococcygeus.

THE PASSENGER: THE BABY

In order to cope with the mechanical stresses and strains of labour, the fetal skull at term is equipped with a highly resilient structure, in the form of non-fused sutures and fontanelles. The degree of movement at these lines, although limited, offers a remarkable reduction in the presenting diameters. The shortest diameter in the fetal skull is the suboccipitobregmatic diameter (average 9.5 cm), with which the vertex presents in the occipitoanterior position. In the occipitoposterior position, the presenting diameter is the occipitofrontal or the suboccipitofrontal (average 11.75 cm and 11 cm respectively). However, in brow presentation, the presenting diameter is the occipitomental (average 13 cm), which generally results in obstructed labour (**Fig. 2.5**).

The general flexion attitude of the fetus, and particularly that of the head, is aided by the presence of efficient uterine contractions, to result in a better mechanical relationship with the pelvis. Efficient uterine contractions, together with the gutter arrangement of the pelvic diaphragm, resolve most malpositions of the fetal head, brought about by poor flexion attitudes, chance or the shape of the pelvic inlet, as in the occipitoposterior position.

During labour, the pelvic cavity is gradually occupied by the fetal head, which distends the vagina; the rectum becomes compressed, as does the bladder under the added pressure of the stretched lower uterine segment, to which it is attached.

THE PELVIC PHASE OF LABOUR

The pelvic phase is that part of labour when full cervical dilatation is approached, and the cardinal movements of the presenting part within the pelvic cavity start to take place. This coincides with the end of the first stage of labour and extends into the second stage.

Friedman described three physiological phases of labour: preparatory, dilatational and pelvic. This must not be confused with descriptions of the first, second and third *stages* of labour. The latter classification relies on fixed end results: full cervical dilatation, delivery of the baby, and delivery of the placenta and membranes respectively. In normal childbirth, the fetus passes through the birth canal in a caudally directed spiral movement, pushed by the pressure of uterine contractions, which maximize the flexion attitude of the fetus. The baby's head negotiates the pelvic cavity either in the transverse diameter of the inlet, or in one of its oblique diameters; in the latter instance, the occiput may be either anteriorly or posteriorly situated.

It is the changing shape and dimension of each part of the pelvis that contribute to the movement of the head within it, and which therefore dictate the extent of rotation required for the delivery of the baby. For the sagittal suture to be aligned with the anteroposterior diameter of the pelvic outlet, the head has to rotate 45° if the occiput is anteriorly situated (**Fig. 2.6a**), 135° if it is posteriorly situated (**Fig. 2.6b**) or 90° if the head enters the pelvis with the sagittal suture in the transverse diameter (**Fig. 2.6c**).

If the fetal head is well flexed, with the occiput anteriorly situated, it rarely experiences any difficulty in negotiating the forwardly directed portion of the cylindrical birth canal. Occasionally, problems may arise if the head enters the lower part of the birth canal in the oblique or transverse position. For delivery to take place, the sagittal plane of the fetal head must align with the anteroposterior diameter of the outlet; this internal rotation of the presenting

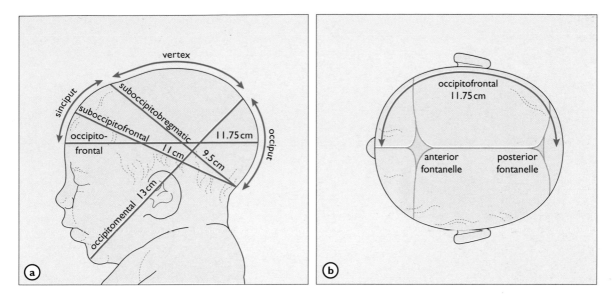

Fig. 2.5a & b The presenting diameters of the fetal skull: **a**, from the side; **b**, from the top.

part is brought about by the uterine contractions and the gutter effect of the levator ani muscle. Failure of the occiput to rotate anteriorly, or its rotation to a direct occipitoposterior position, indicates that the fetal head is poorly flexed and that the degree of deflexion has encouraged the sinciput to move anteriorly (**Fig. 2.7**). The same applies when the occiput persists in the transverse position, although the prominence of the ischial spines does play a part here.

The caudally directed pivot movement of the fetal head within the pelvic cavity aligns the set. Upon further descent, the fetal head is born by extension, with the occiput under the symphysis pubis. After the emergence of the head from the vulva, internal rotation must therefore be reversed (restitution). In order to align the bisacromial diameter with the anteroposterior diameter of the outlet, another internal rotation takes place; from outside, this is seen by the attendant as the external rotation of the head. The anterior shoulder may then be delivered under the symphysis pubis, followed by the posterior shoulder, which clears the posterior vaginal wall and the hollow of the sacrum. The rest of the baby then follows.

If the uterine contractions are efficient enough to result in full cervical dilatation, and to push the presenting part of the fetus into a pelvis of adequate dimensions, an average-sized baby is born with relative ease. However, sometimes this happy picture of normality does not prevail. When labour lingers, a prolonged phase of repeated inefficient contractions will exhaust both mother and baby. Prolonged labour encourages the development of oedema of the pelvic tissues and may affect the anatomical integrity of the organs adjacent to the vagina; it may also jeopardize the oxygen supply to the fetus, resulting in birth asphyxia.

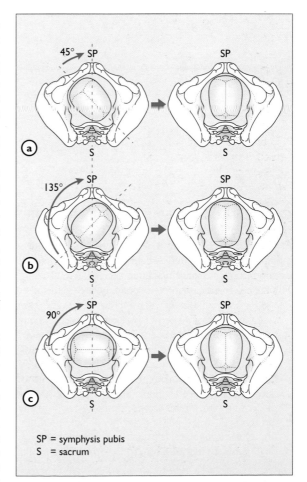

SP = symphysis pubis
S = sacrum

Fig. 2.6a–c Internal rotation of the head: **a**, 45°; **b**, 135°; **c**, 90°.

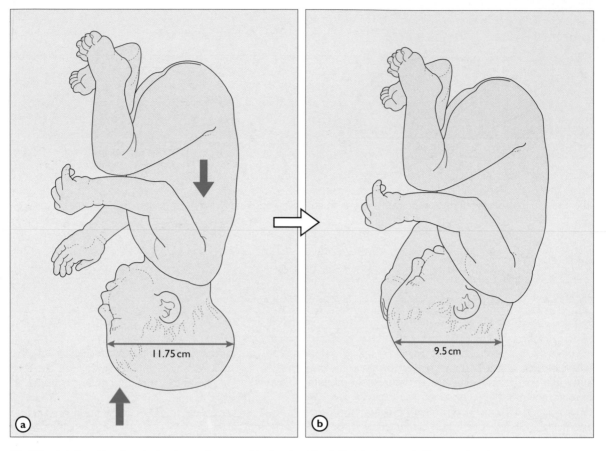
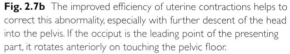

Fig. 2.7a A deflexed head results in a larger diameter of the head presenting to the pelvis.

Fig. 2.7b The improved efficiency of uterine contractions helps to correct this abnormality, especially with further descent of the head into the pelvis. If the occiput is the leading point of the presenting part, it rotates anteriorly on touching the pelvic floor.

CARDINAL MOVEMENTS IN LABOUR

At this stage, it is useful to describe the cardinal movements of the presenting part (in cephalic presentation) during the second stage of labour.

1. *Fetal head descent and increased flexion* are the result of uterine contractions and are usually accomplished, provided that there is no pelvic obstruction caused by bone or soft-tissue pathology, and that the head is of average size. The following movements are all superimposed upon further descent.
2. *Internal rotation* occurs as the presenting part makes contact with the pelvic floor: the leading point of the presenting part rotates to the front as a result of the gutter effect of the pelvic floor. In cephalic presentation, the leading point is usually the occiput, but it can be the sinciput in the deflexed head, which then results in the occipitoposterior position; in breech presentation, the leading point is either the anterior or posterior hip, and in face presentation it is the mentum (chin).

3. *Extension* of the head follows as it reaches the forwardly directed pelvic outlet. The occiput lies under the symphysis pubis and between the pubic rami, which act as a fulcrum. The head is delivered by extension, with the baby's face sweeping the posterior vaginal wall.
4. *Restitution* is the 'undoing' of the internal rotation, and takes place immediately after the emergence of the head from the vulva. It occurs in a direction exactly opposite to that of the internal rotation, and is of the same magnitude.
5. *External rotation* of the head outside the vulva follows restitution, as the shoulders descend onto the pelvic floor; it occurs as the bisacromial diameter is aligned with the anteroposterior diameter of the outlet (another internal rotation). The anterior shoulder appears first under the pubic arch, acting as a fulcrum for the posterior shoulder to be delivered, after this has travelled a longer distance along the posterior vaginal wall. The rest of the baby follows.

Chapter THREE

The Management of Labour

MANAGEMENT OF THE FIRST STAGE OF LABOUR

Much has been written about the management of the first stages of labour; for different approaches to the subject, the interested reader is referred to the works of Friedman, Studd, and O'Driscoll and Meagher.

Labour pain is the only medical condition in which the patient dictates to the attending physician; the diagnosis of labour, the time of her hospital admission and subsequent management. Admission, however, need not necessarily be to the labour ward, where beds are both limited and expensive to maintain and may therefore be given only to those patients in need of them. Whilst labour is defined as the onset of painful uterine contractions of increasing frequency and severity, the final arbiter for the diagnosis of established labour remains progressive cervical dilatation, and therefore it is at this stage that the woman should be admitted to the labour ward.

On admission of the patient to hospital, information is obtained regarding the onset, duration and severity of her uterine contractions, whether a 'show' has been passed, if recent vaginal bleeding or rupture of membranes has occurred, and the presence of other symptoms. The vital signs of pulse, temperature and blood pressure are recorded at this time, and subsequently at hourly intervals during the early part of the first stage of labour.

A general physical examination is performed. The abdomen is examined and the uterine size, fetal presentation and fetal position are recorded. A vaginal examination is conducted to determine the direction of the cervix – whether anterior, posterior or midposition – and the level of the presenting part in relation to the ischial spines, its consistency, the length of the cervical canal, and the dilatation of the cervix (**Fig. 3.1**). When these data are gathered, the examiner sweeps his fingers over the vaginal walls to assess the pelvis and its adequacy. Fetal well-being is also assessed by means of a cardiotocogram (**Fig. 3.2**), which should show accelerations of at least 15 beats/min, lasting for at least 15 seconds, during uterine contractions, fetal movement, or both. At least two such accelerations should be documented within 20 minutes; if not, the cardiography should be continued until this criterion is met.

The findings at the time of hospital admission are assessed, with careful reference to the whole history of the antenatal period and the patient's previous obstetric performance. This information is used to decide whether the patient should be admitted to the labour suite or to the antenatal ward, and whether to proceed with vaginal delivery or otherwise. It is important to emphasize that the

The Bishop score system of assessing changes in the cervix			
	0	1	2
Direction of the cervix	Posterior	Midposition	Anterior
Consistency	Firm	Intermediate	Soft
Application to presenting part	Not applied	Loosely applied	Firmly applied
Length of the cervix	2 cm	1 cm	Effaced
Cervical dilatation	Closed	1–2 cm	3 cm

Fig. 3.1 The Bishop score system of assessing changes in the cervix. After 38 weeks' gestation, the cervix undergoes progressive changes in preparation for labour. These changes include softening of its consistency, and the cervix may sometimes undergo shortening (effacement), or even dilatation of 1–3 cm. In the latent phase of labour, these changes progress further until the active phase of labour is reached, when progressive cervical dilatation occurs. The scoring system shown here, the Bishop score, has been devised to document these changes. The maximum score is 10 when labour enters its active phase; scoring of the cervix on admission of the parturient to the labour ward is a useful guide for diagnosis and subsequent assessments.

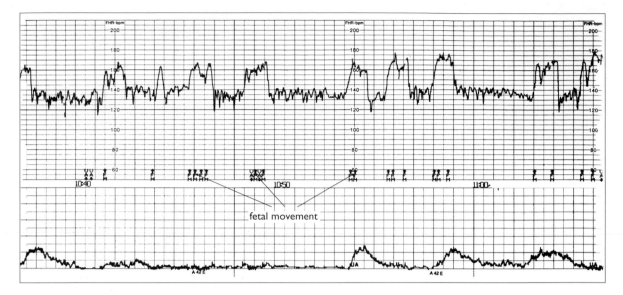

fetal movement

Fig. 3.2 Cardiotocogram in early labour, showing good fetal heart variability and accelerations.

physiological definition of the onset of labour bears only a temporal relationship to the management of the active phase of progressive cervical dilatation, and descent of the presenting part.

If the diagnosis of labour is made, the findings are recorded on a partogram (**Fig. 3.3**); simpler forms also are in use in other hospitals. The appropriate fetal monitoring technique is instituted, whether intermittent auscultation or continuous electronic monitoring of the fetal heart. Whichever form of documentation is followed, progressive cervical dilatation must be confirmed, and any sign of slow progress diagnosed, as early as is practicable. In the labour ward in most obstetric units, a chart is displayed showing a series of circles ranging from 1 to 10 cm in diameter; this helps juniors to interpret the extent of cervical dilatation. Should an abnormality be suspected, a vaginal examination at 3-hourly intervals, or more frequently, is widely acceptable. In fact, when this system is followed, fewer vaginal examinations are performed per labour, as pathological labours may be identified and treated early, whereas those with normal progress infrequently require more than three such examinations.

In addition to assessment of the progress of cervical dilatation, vaginal examination in labour is performed to establish the descent of the head, and whether caput succedaneum or moulding has developed. It is sometimes difficult to assess the position of the fetal head when vaginal examination is performed during labour, particularly when labour has been endured long enough for caput succedaneum and moulding of the skull bones to develop and obscure most of the landmarks. It is therefore always prudent to perform an abdominal examination at the

outset – a manoeuvre that will help to interpret the findings at subsequent vaginal examination. The basic steps during vaginal examination, when assessing the fetal head, are to locate the sagittal suture and, if possible, the anterior fontanelle; as a rule of thumb, a palpable fontanelle is the anterior fontanelle.

If the diagnosis of labour is not made, the findings must be clearly documented; vague terms such as false labour, latent labour, establishing labour and effacing cervix serve only to confuse the patient, the doctors and the midwives. The examination findings should be communicated to the patient in a straightforward, non-technical language, after which she is transferred to the antenatal ward, where ambulation or a hot bath may allay her anxieties and help pass the time until the onset of the active phase of labour, when management will be conducted in the delivery suite. If the patient is tired and keen to sleep, she can be helped with a small dose of sedative or a hypnotic. In a significant number of cases, these 'labour pains' settle down, and provided there is no clinical evidence to suggest placental abruption, and the fetal heart rate tracing is satisfactory, the patient can be sent home the next day.

Women in established labour vary to a large extent in their pain threshold, the extremes being those who quietly reach full cervical dilatation, and those who look completely exhausted with mild contractions of short duration. The majority, however, can cope reasonably well during the early part of the first stage of labour, although they may later require some form of analgesia, such as pethidine or even epidural anaesthesia. Other techniques are sometimes used, such as a paracervical block. Resources permitting,

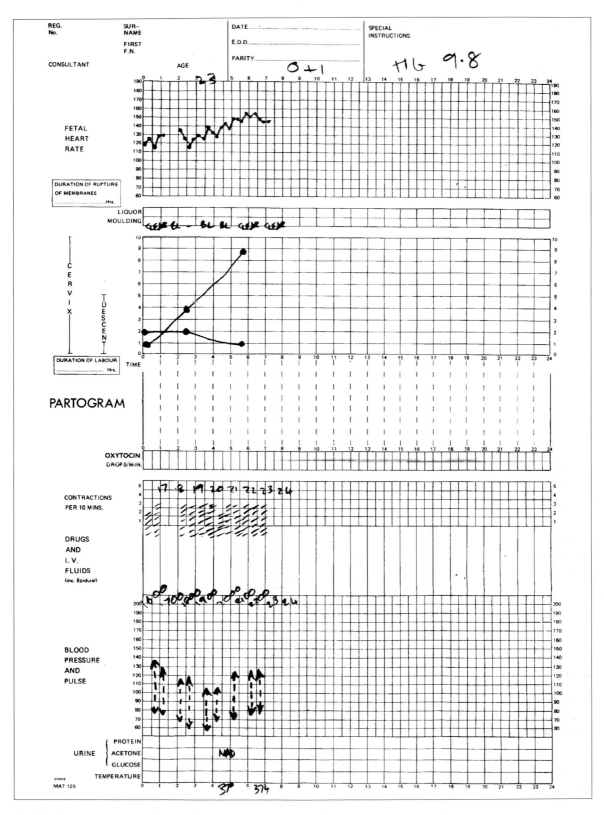

Fig. 3.3 Partogram is a composite chart that includes the patient's identification and helps to present the progress in labour pictorially, in addition to providing recordings of maternal vital signs, fetal heart rate and any medications administered during labour.

it is important to respect the patient's wishes regarding pain relief, as the whole experience of labour may otherwise fall short of her expectations.

It has been customary to ensure that patients in established labour refrain from eating and drinking even clear fluids, in view of the delayed gastric emptying that prevails during pregnancy and, in a more pronounced form, during labour. However, this may not be necessary, especially in early labours in which no clinical problem has been identified in the mother or the baby. If she so desires, in these circumstances a slice of bread and a cup of tea may help the mother, but in advanced labours clear fluids should be advised and will reduce the incidence of dehydration and ketone bodies formation.

A number of studies have investigated the rate of progress in labour. In order to construct a plan for decision-making during the management of the first stage of labour, it is necessary to put the results of these studies in perspective. The main conclusion is that the mean duration of the observed first stage of spontaneous labour is about 6 hours in the primigravida, compared with about 4.5 hours in the multigravida. In addition, the first stage of spontaneous labour takes less than 10 hours in 88% of primigravidae, compared with 95% of multigravidae. Cervical dilatation at the rate of 1 cm/hour therefore represents the slowest rate of acceptable normal progress in labour. Failure to achieve full cervical dilatation within these time limits, especially after the stage of a 6-cm dilated cervix, should alert the attendant to the possibility of cephalopelvic disproportion, whether it be absolute, due to the fetal head lying in the occipitoposterior position or, more commonly, the result of inefficient uterine contractions.

There have been a number of attempts at introducing a pressure catheter to measure intrauterine pressure as an index of 'adequate uterine contraction'. The technique remains a research tool, and its practicability has not been widely accepted. There are many cases on record of uterine rupture and uterine scar dehiscence in units where intrauterine pressure monitoring is used routinely; in some cases, the incidents went unnoticed until the time of caesarean section. There is no evidence that the incidence of uterine rupture, maternal or perinatal morbidity or mortality is any lower when intrauterine pressure catheters are in routine use. The alternative and pragmatic approach, which has stood the test of time, is that described by O'Driscoll and Meagher. This approach is based on the concept of the early diagnosis of labour, monitoring by frequency and duration of uterine contractions, by palpation or by tocographic recording, the supervision of adequate cervimetric progress and the early diagnosis of abnormal labour, and, equally importantly, the provision of one midwife to attend that labour. Their policy has resulted in a healthy rate of normal deliveries, and in the lowest rate of caesarean sections in Western Europe, with comparable success as regards perinatal mortality and morbidity.

INDUCTION OF LABOUR

Interruption of the course of pregnancy may be indicated in a number of conditions when it is judged that continuation of pregnancy may pose a greater risk to maternal or fetal well-being. The common indications for induction of labour include pre-eclampsia, intrauterine growth retardation and the continuation of a pregnancy beyond 42 weeks. The principle that governs successful induction of labour is the initiation of rhythmic uterine contractions that will induce effacement and dilatation of the cervix. This can be achieved by amniotomy (see below), or rupture of membranes, followed by infusion of oxytocin. The process can be facilitated by prior vaginal administration of prostaglandin E2 in a gel form, which helps to soften the cervix and stimulate uterine contractions, and which in turn induces further cervical ripening and dilatation. Amniotomy is performed when the cervix is 3 cm dilated or more, and is usually followed by active labour. Another approach is to insert a finger into the cervix and separate the fetal membrane from the lower segment (sweeping the membranes), which may result in the release of local prostaglandins. However, it may cause undue discomfort and is not as effective as previous techniques.

AMNIOTOMY

Rupture of the membranes occurs spontaneously during the first stage of labour, especially close to full dilatation of the cervix. Artificial rupture of the membranes (amniotomy) increases the frequency and strength of uterine contractions and is usually performed to induce labour or to accelerate it, should the first stage be slow, particularly during the second half of the first stage of labour. Amniotomy is conducted by vaginal examination, where the amniohook is guided by the examining fingers to the forewaters (the bag of fetal membranes), which leads ahead of the presenting part (**Figs 3.4 & 3.5**). It is wise to obtain a recording of the fetal heart by cardiotocography for the following 20 minutes.

FETAL SCALP BLOOD SAMPLING

During the course of labour, concern may arise regarding fetal well-being. As a result of this, fetal scalp blood sampling (**Figs 3.6–3.9**) has been developed, and is attracting a great deal of interest amongst obstetricians, many of whom have adopted this technique as an integral part of routine monitoring in labour.

Indications for the use of this invasive technique can be summarized in two categories: when fetal heart tracing is suggestive of fetal acidosis; or when fresh meconium-stained liquor appears *per vaginam*. The results must be interpreted carefully. A pH value less than 7.20 indicates delivery by the abdominal route or, in suitable cases, by operative vaginal delivery. The latter course can be followed in the case of full dilatation of the cervix with the head low down in the pelvis, especially in a rapidly progressing labour. If the fetal scalp blood pH is greater than 7.25, it is reasonable to exclude acidosis, but if values lie

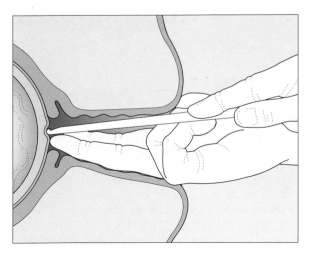

Fig. 3.4 Amniotomy.

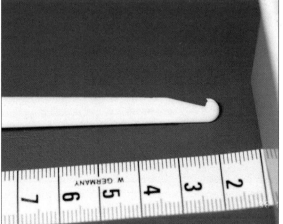

Fig. 3.5 A plastic amniohook in common use.

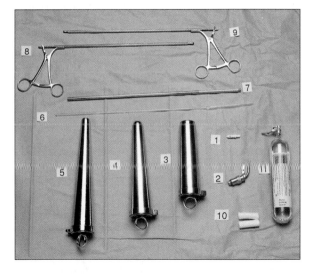

Fig. 3.6 The instruments required in fetal scalp blood sampling:
1   A 2-mm deep blade (see **Fig. 3.9**).
2   Light head (see **Fig. 3.7**).
3–5   Amnioscopes.
6   Capillary tube.
7   Blade handle.
8&9   Swab holders.
10   Dental rolls (cotton).
11   Ethyl chloride.

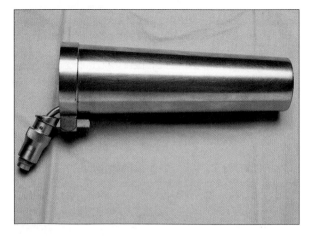

Fig. 3.7 Fetal scalp blood sampling: a large-sized amnioscope, illuminated with a fibreoptic lead.

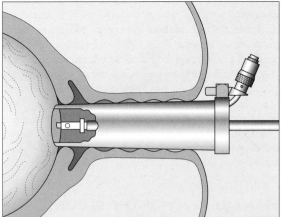

Fig. 3.8 The amnioscope is introduced into the vagina, guided into the cervix by the examiner's fingers, and pressed against the presenting part. The fetal scalp is stabbed with the blade.

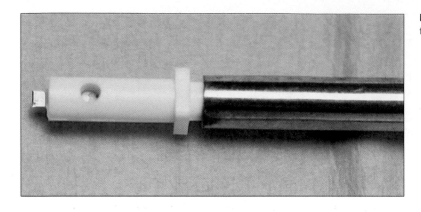

Fig. 3.9 A close-up view of the blade used for fetal blood sampling

between 7.20 and 7.25, the sampling must be repeated within 30 minutes, if the fetal heart tracing suggests that such a wait is permissible. It is essential to consult the original work of Saling, and to look at the normal distribution of the pH values and how they correlate with the outcome of labour. The reproducibility of pH measurements must be carefully interpreted in relation to the variability of the sample collection and the coefficient of variation of the machine in use.

New developments in percutaneous oximeters have produced probes that can be fitted on the fetal scalp and coupled to fetal scalp electrodes to produce simultaneous readings. Controlled clinical trials are required before these techniques can be introduced into routine clinical practice. After all, intrapartum hypoxia is only one of the many causes of mental and physical handicap, and genetic and other environmental factors must not be overlooked.

Technique

The patient is usually placed in the lithotomy position, with a wedge under her right side, but the procedure can also be performed with the parturient in the left lateral position.

The fetal scalp is cleaned with cotton rolls, sprayed with ethyl chloride, and a high-vacuum silicone grease is applied. Ethyl chloride will help to arterialize the scalp tissue by inducing reactive vasodilatation, whilst the high pressure silicone grease will help the blood released from the scalp to form a droplet, thus assisting aspiration. The fetal scalp is then stabbed with a small, 2-mm deep blade (**Fig. 3.9**), and the blood drops collected in heparinized capillary pipettes. Gentle suction must be applied, lest air bubbles are sucked into the tube, invalidating the reading of the blood pH value.

MANAGEMENT OF THE SECOND STAGE OF LABOUR

The second stage of labour is the expulsive phase; it starts when the cervix becomes fully dilated and continues until delivery of the baby. Its average duration in spontaneous uncomplicated labours is about 40 minutes in the primigravida and 15 minutes in the multiparous woman. Failure to achieve the delivery of the child within these time limits does not necessarily indicate operative delivery, but does demand a reappraisal of the situation regarding the position or size of the fetus in relation to the pelvis. In women who have had an effective epidural block, the fetal head is often seen to be lying low down in the pelvis, resting on the perineum, but no further advance is achieved, as the mother's urge to push has been obtunded.

Provided that the position of the fetus is carefully ascertained and the head is lying in the occipitoanterior position, in the absence of marked caput or significant moulding, the second stage can be allowed to continue for a little longer. When there is no sign of serious fetal heart decelerations, or of hypoxia and acidosis, there is no harm in waiting for the return of the mother's urge to bear down, in order to deliver the baby.

However, delaying the delivery far beyond 1 hour in the second stage should be allowed only after an experienced obstetrician has carefully assessed the situation. This is particularly true when the duration of the latter part of the first stage of labour – the stage between 7-cm and full dilatation of the cervix – is more than 3 hours. It is necessary to examine such patients carefully and request an experienced person to review the course of labour.

It is emphasized that today's obstetricians must not regard full cervical dilatation as the point of no return, or delivery of the child *per vaginam* as a challenge to their manual dexterity.

EPISIOTOMY

The word 'episiotomy' literally means 'cutting of the pudenda or genitals'; the operation to which this term is applied, however, is in fact a perineotomy, or an incision of the perineum. An episiotomy involves a small surgical incision into the perineum, which helps to protect the posterior vulval tissue and the perineal muscles from suffering excessive distension by the fetal head, and replaces a ragged vaginal and perineal tear with neat, clean-cut tissue that is more likely to be repaired satisfactorily. It also helps to reduce the resistance against the advancing presenting part, hence its recommendation in the birth of premature babies.

In each of its three forms – median, posterolateral and mediolateral – episiotomy achieves the same objective, but the immediate complications and future sequelae differ. Median episiotomy is associated with loss of a smaller amount of blood, easier repair and much less pain during healing than is posterolateral episiotomy. However, median episiotomy carries a high risk of extension into the rectum. Mediolateral episiotomy (**Fig. 3.10**) offers an acceptable compromise. Most operators use a pair of scissors to perform the operation, although, in experienced hands, a scalpel can produce neat and well-controlled incisions.

It is important to appreciate that episiotomy is not a mandatory accompaniment of operative deliveries. A well-controlled delivery of the head in spontaneous labour, or even with forceps or ventouse (vacuum extraction), can be accomplished without episiotomy in many suitable cases. The least trauma and easiest repair are achieved when a timely episiotomy is performed – that is, when the presenting part distends the vulva. A poorly controlled delivery of the head, however, results in a number of ragged tears of the vagina, perineum and vulva, despite the performance of an episiotomy.

MANAGEMENT OF THE THIRD STAGE OF LABOUR

The third stage of labour is that of placental separation, which begins after the baby is born and ends with the delivery of the placenta and fetal membranes.

During pregnancy, the placenta is anchored to the uterine wall by innumerable capillaries and supportive tissues that invade the uterus. The anchoring villi are bathed in a pool of maternal blood that amounts to 100–150 ml.

The sudden decompression of the uterine cavity following the delivery of the baby results in the contraction and retraction of the uterine muscle. This produces a discrepancy between the uterine surface and the non-contracting placenta, and this discrepancy, in turn, places a great shearing force on the attaching fibres, resulting in their breakage. The contraction of the uterine muscle fibres acts as a tourniquet to the intervening blood vessels and leads to the closure of the uterine venules; the pool of maternal blood bathing the placenta is consequently prevented from being injected back into the maternal circulation. This blood places added weight behind the placenta, to effect further separation of the membranes attached to the lower parts of the uterus. The appearance of a gush of blood *per vaginam* therefore heralds the separation of the placenta. In addition, as the placenta clears the upper parts

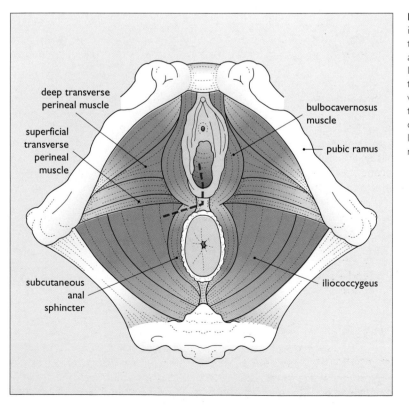

deep transverse perineal muscle

superficial transverse perineal muscle

subcutaneous anal sphincter

bulbocavernosus muscle

pubic ramus

iliococcygeus

Fig. 3.10 Mediolateral episiotomy: the incision is indicated by the dotted line, and the muscles through which it is performed are shown. Note that support for the lateral part of the pelvic floor is maintained through its attachment to the bony pelvis, whilst the medial part has no such support; this is the main reason why the medial edge of the vaginal wound looks longer than the lateral edge, once the incision has been made.

of the uterus, the fundus is seen to rise and to become narrow and more globular, and the cord lengthens.

In assisting the delivery of the placenta, it is wise not to proceed by massaging the uterine fundus, or by attempting to push the uterus into the pelvis; this only causes pain and discomfort to the patient and risks the development of acute uterine inversion. Controlled cord traction is a far safer technique, whereby the placenta is pulled through traction on the cord, whilst the uterus is held and directed posteriorly and cephalad (towards the head).

Meddlesome practices to expedite the delivery of the placenta often result in inco-ordinate uterine contraction and delay the delivery of the placenta, through the inducement of a ring of contraction below it, or the cord may be snapped due to excessive traction.

After its delivery, the placenta is inspected for completeness, and the umbilical cord is examined so that the number of vessels may be noted. The uterus is palpated *per abdomen*, and its firmness and the level of its fundus are recorded.

Chapter FOUR

Pain Relief in Labour

Labour pain is unique compared with other forms of acute pain. It has a very wide range of severity, hence views about the need for its relief are very diverse. Even the extreme pain of labour is often forgotten after the baby's arrival, leaving behind a vivid memory of the side-effects of the method of pain relief (minor though they may be).

Pain relief in labour is provided to minimize the deleterious effects of stress on the mother and the baby. There are various methods of pain relief, the choice among which is influenced by: first, the availability, at the place of delivery, of both the method itself and staff appropriately skilled in its use; second, the wishes of the mother, which are conditioned by the information given to her during preparation for childbirth; third, any co-existing medical condition; and finally, and perhaps most importantly, the nature of the obstetric process and the intervention. Consideration of the effects of analgesia on the baby is of paramount importance.

Several methods of pain relief are available, but none possesses all the attributes of the ideal agent, which must be safe, simple to administer and effective. Personal care given continuously during labour by the midwife reduces any fear, anxiety and loneliness that may be experienced by the parturient, and may eliminate the need for many complicated techniques. Psychological techniques – hypnosis, breathing exercises, transcutaneous electrical nerve stimulation (TENS) – are also available, and have been used with limited degrees of success.

NITROUS OXIDE

The most commonly used inhalation agent is nitrous oxide (N_2O). It is always used with oxygen, in the form of a compressed gas mixture (1 : 1) delivered by the Entonox apparatus. This consists of a portable cylinder containing the premixed gases, a reducing valve, a demand valve having a very low resistance to breathing, a cylinder contents gauge and a corrugated hose connected to a face-mask; the face-mask may be replaced by a disposable mouthpiece. To obtain effective analgesia, the mother is instructed to start inhaling the gas at the first moment when she feels a contraction, and not to wait until it becomes painful. The cycle is repeated with each contraction.

The advantage of nitrous oxide over other inhalation agents is that it has no cumulative effect and therefore, theoretically, there is no limitation to the duration for which it may be administered in labour. In addition, it has the advantage of containing 50% oxygen, which is beneficial to the fetus. It is usually given during the late part of the first stage of labour, when another dose of a narcotic analgesic is to be avoided, and in the second stage of labour.

SYSTEMIC ANALGESICS

In the United Kingdom, 38% of women in labour are given pethidine, which has taken precedence in the list of narcotic analgesics to be administered in labour for the past 50 years. A 100-mg dose of pethidine given intramuscularly produces satisfactory pain relief in 10% of labouring women; 150 mg helps pain relief in 50–60% of these women, but becomes associated with more side-effects. Pethidine has one advantage over morphine, namely its greater lipid solubility, giving it a rapid onset of action; its only advantage over epidural analgesia is that it is readily available.

Unpleasant side-effects of pethidine include nausea, vomiting, drowsiness and disorientation; a more serious side-effect is delay in gastric emptying.

Seventy per cent of the concentration of pethidine in maternal blood is detectable in the fetus, as a result of placental transfer. Pethidine has active metabolites that accumulate slowly in the fetal tissue; this explains the high incidence of fetal ventilatory depression when repeated doses of pethidine are given to the mother. Opioid-induced neonatal ventilatory depression can be reversed by naloxone, which is a pure narcotic antagonist, but if a mother who has received repeated doses of pethidine requires further pain relief and delivery of the infant is not imminent, consideration should be given to the use of a more effective, albeit invasive, analgesic technique.

EPIDURAL ANALGESIA

Pain during the first stage of labour is caused by uterine contractions and cervical dilatation, pain impulses entering the spinal cord at the T10, T11, T12 and L1 spinal segments. Pain experienced late in the first stage and during the second stage of labour is caused by stretching of the pelvic floor muscles and the perineum; these pain impulses travel via the pudendal nerves and enter the spinal cord at the level of the S2, S3 and S4 spinal segments. Effective epidural analgesia for labour pain thus requires a sensory block extending from T10 to S5, with minimal motor block.

Epidural analgesia is the most effective method of pain relief in labour; nevertheless, it is an invasive technique and requires skilled medical and nursing staff to manage it. It produces excellent and continuous pain relief in more than 70% of patients. Compared with other methods of pain relief, epidural analgesia produces fewer changes in the biochemical environments of the fetus and the mother, as it abolishes the hyperventilation, and hence hypocapnoea, associated with pain and apprehension. In addition, metabolic acidosis is less severe than that associated with pethidine. Not surprisingly, therefore, the use of epidural analgesia is increasing in most maternity units in the United Kingdom; in the USA, the rate of use of the technique is approximately 50%.

Epidural analgesia is indicated in labour for pain relief regardless of the degree of cervical dilatation, on request by the parturient. Many maternity units consider certain obstetric conditions to be indications for epidural analgesia; these include pregnancy-induced hypertension, pre-eclampsia without coagulopathy, trial of scar, breech presentation, twins, preterm labour and any medical condition in which sympathoadrenal overactivity is undesirable. Unfortunately, there are some contraindications to the use of epidural analgesia, including refusal by the mother, coagulopathy, local infection at the site of insertion of the epidural catheter, untreated hypovolaemia and increased intracranial pressure. The risk of regional anaesthesia in HIV-positive patients has been evaluated in a small number of such patients; the results suggest that regional anaesthesia can be safely performed in this group.

Technique

Before the epidural block is embarked upon, an intravenous cannula should be put in place. Most anaesthetists prefer to have the patient in the lateral lumbar puncture position, although the sitting position is preferred by others, because it provides better lumbar flexion and a better view of the landmarks (**Fig. 4.1**).

The mother sits on the edge of the bed with her back flexed. Through a sterile towel, under completely aseptic conditions, the iliac crests are palpated; the L4–L5 interspace is located at this level. The L3–L4 or L2–L3 interspace is usually chosen for access to the epidural space. By means of a 25G needle, a skin weal is raised at the interspace chosen and the subcutaneous tissue is infiltrated with a local anaesthetic solution (1% lignocaine hydrochloride). To facilitate the insertion of the blunt-ended Tuohy needle (16G or 18G), the skin is nicked, either with a scalpel blade or, even better, with the sharp, bevelled edge of an ordinary injection needle, to avoid introducing a plug of skin into the epidural space. The Tuohy needle is inserted with a steady, controlled pressure, its bevel pointing upwards, and passed through the subcutaneous tissue and supraspinous ligament. Now the stylet is withdrawn and a 10-ml syringe, filled with air or sterile saline, is attached to the needle. The hub of the needle is grasped firmly by the thumb and index finger of the left hand, and the other fingers rest against the patient's back, to ensure maximum control of the needle; the thumb of the right hand keeps a

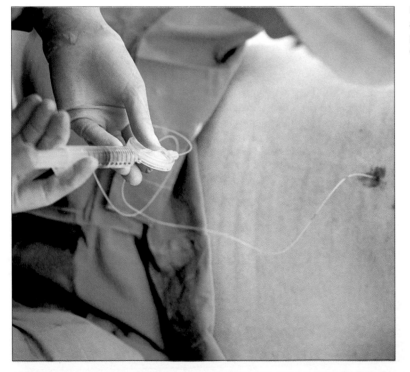

Fig. 4.1a Administration of epidural anaesthesia: the patient is in the sitting position at the edge of the bed, with an epidural catheter *in situ*.

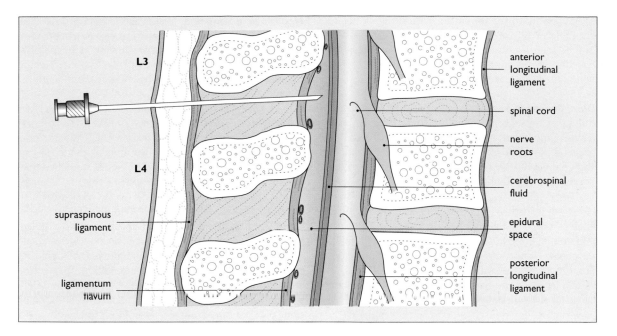

L3

L4

anterior
longitudinal
ligament

spinal cord

nerve
roots

cerebrospinal
fluid

epidural
space

posterior
longitudinal
ligament

supraspinous
ligament

ligamentum
flavum

Fig. 4.1b Administration of epidural anaesthesia: the Tuohy needle is in the epidural space.

constant moderate pressure on the plunger of the syringe. Using the left hand only, the needle is slowly and steadily advanced through the interspinous ligament. When the ligamentum flavum is approached, the resistance increases. This is followed by a sudden loss of resistance when the needle reaches the epidural space, and the advance of the needle must then be stopped.

The use of air to identify the epidural space is not without problems, and it has been reported to cause incomplete analgesia, unblocked segments, air embolus and an associated high incidence of dural tap. Dural tap is one of the complications of epidural analgesia that must not be overlooked. If an air-filled syringe has been used, any fluid that issues through the needle after the syringe has been disconnected must be cerebrospinal fluid (CSF). In the case of a saline-filled syringe being used, if more than a few drops of liquid flow back from the hub of the needle, a dural puncture must be suspected. If aspiration through the needle produces a continuous flow of fluid, a dural puncture is confirmed.

For a continuous epidural block technique, an epidural catheter is inserted through the needle and advanced. When it enters the epidural space, a slight resistance is felt; at that point, a further 5 cm of the catheter is introduced and the needle is slid over the catheter by maintaining pressure on the catheter during withdrawal. Now the catheter is securely fixed to the skin at the point of entry, by means of waterproof adhesive tape. The standard practice is to use a bacterial filter, both as a precaution against infection and to trap any glass particles from the broken ampoules that contained the local anaesthetic. Aspiration of the catheter should be performed, to exclude dural puncture by the catheter or

intravascular placement of the catheter, after which a test-dose of 3 ml of 2% lignocaine is given. When the local anaesthetic is inadvertently injected into the subarachnoid space, its neural block becomes manifest within a short time. Therefore, 5 minutes after the test-dose is administered, if the patient is able to move her toes without a tingling sensation, a subarachnoid injection of the local anaesthetic may be reasonably excluded.

Bupivacaine is the local anaesthetic of choice for continuous epidural analgesia because of its long duration of action and low fetal : maternal concentration ratio. In the past, 0.375–0.5% bupivacaine was widely used, as intermittent bolus doses to a total volume of 8–10 ml. Currently, more dilute solutions of local anaesthetic are used, to maintain motor power. A total dose of 2 mg/kg body weight should not be exceeded.

During epidural blocks, the blood pressure should be monitored every 1–2 minutes for the first 10 minutes after the injection of local anaesthetic, and then every 5–10 minutes until the block wears off. The mother must not be left unattended, and should always be managed in the lateral position, to reduce aortocaval compression. If unilateral analgesia occurs, the patient is turned on her other side, and more local anaesthetic is injected (5 ml).

Complications
Hypotension. This remains the most common side-effect of regional anaesthesia. Its severity and frequency depend on the extent of the block, the position of the mother and her blood volume. Prophylactic measures include intravenous fluid loading before the block, and use of the

lateral position to minimize aortocaval occlusion. Hypotension is treated by the intravenous administration of fluid, and if normal blood pressure is not regained, ephedrine 3–5 mg is given intravenously. Close observation of the fetal heart must be maintained.

Dural Puncture. The incidence of accidental dural puncture varies with the experience of the anaesthetist; in the hands of the expert, it should be less than 0.5%. If dural puncture is recognized, the needle should be withdrawn and epidural block performed at an adjacent interspace. Because of the high incidence (70–80%) of severe headaches after unintentional dural puncture, it should be actively treated, as follows. *a*: After delivery, the catheter is left *in situ* and a sterile Ringer's lactate solution is slowly infused into the epidural space over the next 24 hours; *b*: the patient is encouraged to stay in bed, in the prone position if possible, for 24 hours; *c*: regular simple analgesic should be given, and high fluid intake should be encouraged; *d*: if these measures are not effective, an experienced anaesthetist should insert a blood patch into the epidural space under sterile conditions and the mother should be advised to lie supine for 2 hours and to avoid straining and back movements for 2 weeks. In the presence of pyrexia, autologous blood patching is contraindicated, because of the risk of bacteraemia and the formation of an epidural abscess. An alternative method of treating postdural puncture headache is the intravenous infusion of caffeine.

Total Spinal Anaesthesia. This is caused by inadvertent subarachnoid injection of the full dose of local anaesthetic, and is characterized by hypotension, ascending paralysis of the legs, trunk and ventilatory muscles, and apnoea. Hypotension should be treated as described above, and an airway should be established and the lungs ventilated with oxygen. If necessary, endotracheal intubation should be performed, to protect the airway from aspiration.

Toxic Reaction. This may occur as the result of accidental intravascular injection of the local anaesthetic or the injection of an overdose of local anaesthetic into the epidural space. Symptoms such as tinnitus, drowsiness and disorientation may precede generalized convulsions, which may cease before an anticonvulsant drug is given. The airway should be maintained and oxygen should be administered. Diazepam is given to control convulsions, but, if these persist, thiopentone should be administered by intravenous injection.

Bupivacaine is cardiotoxic in high doses, causing arrhythmias followed by cardiac depression and arrest. These should be treated appropriately by external cardiac massage, defibrillation if necessary, intravenous fluid, and ionotropic drugs when required. Uterine displacement should be maintained.

Neurological Sequelae. Significant neurological damage after vertebral blocks is very rare. Damage to a nerve root by a needle or catheter, or from pressure by a foreign body, and arachnoiditis resulting from chemical contamination or infection have been reported. Other complications include infected epidural haematomas.

Neurological sequelae cannot be attributed solely to regional block, because obstetric injuries in the absence of regional block are also well recognized. These include pressure by the fetal head or the forceps blade on the nerves of lumbosacral plexus. Another obstetric mechanism for neurological complication is ischaemic damage to the lower spinal cord caused by the fetal head if it occludes the arterial supply. Coincidental acute disc lesion during labour may contribute to some cases. Postnatal backache associated with regional analgesia has been concluded to be the result of the combination of motor blockade, good analgesia and bad posture. Recent prospective studies with long-term follow-up have shown no difference in the incidence of new backache between populations that did or did not receive epidural analgesia.

CAUDAL ANALGESIA

With the availability of epidural lumbar analgesia, caudal analgesia has not been favoured, particularly in the first stage of labour. It is used mainly in the second stage of labour, for forceps delivery, as it produces a more rapid onset of perineal analgesia and muscle relaxation than does epidural block.

Technique

The aseptic technique that is used for epidural block should also be applied to caudal analgesia. The sacral cornua that lie on either side of the hiatus are palpated, local anaesthetic solution is used to make a skin weal at the sacral hiatus, and the subcutaneous tissue is infiltrated (**Fig. 4.2**).

At an angle of 70° to the skin, a short-bevel caudal needle is inserted through the skin and the sacrococcygeal membrane that covers the sacral hiatus. When this membrane has been pierced, the hub of the needle is depressed until it makes an angle of 20° with the skin. The needle is advanced in the sacral canal by not more than 2 cm, to avoid puncturing the dural sac, and an aspiration test for CSF or blood is made. If blood is aspirated, the needle should be withdrawn 0.5 cm and the test repeated. If CSF is withdrawn, the procedure should be abandoned or converted to one of subarachnoid block. A test-dose of 3 ml of local anaesthetic is injected in the sacral canal and this should not be met with resistance if the needle is correctly placed. After 5 minutes, the mother should be asked if she can move her toes (see explanation in Epidural Analgesia section on page 36). For pain relief in the first stage of labour, a total of 20 ml of local anaesthetic is required; 0.25%

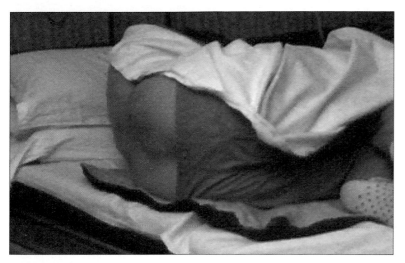

Fig. 4.2a Caudal analgesia: the patient assumes the left lateral position, in preparation for the caudal block.

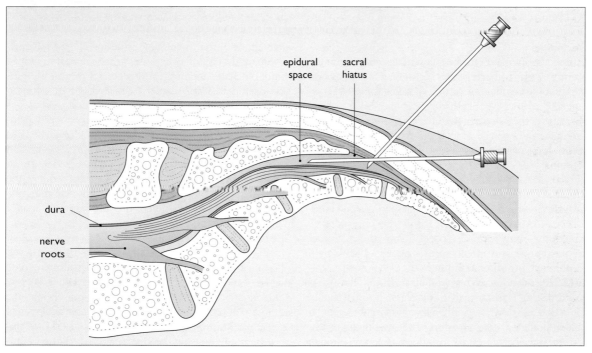

epidural space   sacral hiatus

dura

nerve roots

Fig. 4.2b Caudal analgesia: the needle is manipulated into the epidural space.

bupivacaine is preferred, to avoid administration of a large dose. For second stage pain relief, 10 ml is required. Continuous caudal analgesia can be provided using an epidural catheter, which can be inserted into the sacral canal through a 16G or 18G caudal needle.

Complications
Complications of caudal analgesia are similar to those associated with lumbar epidural block. In addition, the technique carries a risk of injection of a relatively large dose of local anaesthetic into the fetus, which may result in fetal death. There are also the risks associated with the use of a large dose of local anaesthetic, when the technique is used to relieve first stage pains and a large volume is required.

Caudal analgesia may be more difficult to perform than epidural lumbar block, even in experienced hands. This is because of the high incidence of anatomical abnormalities of the sacrum, obesity and oedema, which make it difficult to locate anatomical landmarks.

SPINAL ANALGESIA

If epidural analgesia has not been requested early in labour and operative vaginal delivery or manual removal of the placenta is subsequently indicated, a spinal block may be required, in view of its rapid onset of action, intense analgesia, marked motor block (favoured in rotational forceps delivery and caesarean section) and advantage of requiring only a small dose of local anaesthetic.

A saddle block is used for outlet forceps delivery; as only the sacral roots are blocked (analgesia is limited to the perineal skin and vagina), motor block and other complications are avoided. Saddle block is achieved with a hyperbaric spinal solution of less than 1 ml, administered while the mother is in a sitting position, which she maintains for 3 minutes.

Low spinal block produces analgesia that is adequate for rotational forceps delivery and manual removal of the placenta. With this technique, the block should extend to T10.

Technique

Aseptic technique should be followed meticulously, in the same way as for other regional blocks. An intravenous cannula should be put in place, and a loading volume of crystalloid fluid is advised. The patient assumes either a sitting or a lateral position; although the position of the patient may affect the spread of local anaesthetic, the extent of the block is not predictable, and this is one disadvantage of spinal block. A skin weal is raised over the 3rd or 4th lumbar space. A fine-bore, non-cutting spinal needle is used (25G or 26G), to reduce the incidence and severity of postspinal headache, but necessitates the use of an introducer. A 19G needle can be used for this purpose, provided that only 2 cm is inserted into the skin and supraspinous and interspinous ligaments. The spinal needle is introduced through the 19G needle and advanced steadily. When the ligamentum flavum is pierced, a high resistance to the needle is felt, and it should be advanced slowly for only a few more millimetres, at which point it pierces the dura. The stylet is then withdrawn. It may be necessary to perform aspiration through the needle to confirm that it is in the subarachnoid space, as free flow of CSF would not be expected to occur through a small needle; local anaesthetic should not be injected before the CSF has been identified. If blood is aspirated, the needle should be withdrawn and the puncture repeated at another spinal interspace. If injection of the local anaesthetic is accompanied by any discomfort, the injection should be stopped immediately, to avoid damage to the nerve root or spinal cord.

Complications

Hypotension is caused by preganglionic sympathetic block resulting in vasodilatation and reduction in venous return to the heart. Its severity depends on the extent of the spinal block; it may be accompanied by bradycardia. *Inadvertent high spinal block* may result in ventilatory paralysis and apnoea. Treatment of these complications is described in the section on epidural analgesia.

Postspinal Headache. The incidence of post-dural puncture headache is related to the size of dural hole caused by the spinal needle. This type of headache is believed to be due to a decrease in CSF pressure secondary to CSF leakage as a result of dural puncture. Neurological complications such as paraplegia and transient paraesthesia have been reported, but they are extremely rare. They are caused by mechanical damage to the spinal cord or nerve roots, and chemical or infectious arachnoiditis.

NEW TRENDS IN EPIDURAL DRUGS AND TECHNIQUES

For a long time, the increase in the number of instrumental and operative deliveries has been attributed to the intensity of motor block associated with the use of concentrated local anaesthetics given epidurally. Consequently, various adaptations of the traditional technique of epidural analgesia have developed over recent years, in order to reduce motor blockade and improve analgesia. Continuous infusion of diluted bupivacaine (0.0625–0.125%) using an infusion pump produces consistent analgesia and reduces both the need for top-ups and the number of hypotensive episodes. Patient-controlled epidural analgesia (PCEA) with a combination of bupivacaine (0.1–0.125%) and an opioid, usually fentanyl (1–2 μg/ml), is used widely nowadays in the United Kingdom. This method reduces the requirement for bupivacaine by 50%, thus also minimizing motor block and hypotension, and improves maternal satisfaction and expulsive effort.

The combined technique of intrathecal injection of an opioid and insertion of an epidural catheter has been developed recently, to improve analgesia and maintain some degree of mobility in labour – hence the names 'mobile epidural' or 'walking epidural'. This technique also has the advantage of producing rapid onset of reliable analgesia of as much as 3 hours' duration. Thereafter, analgesia is maintained epidurally using the combination of diluted bupivacaine and fentanyl. However, with this method it seems that respiratory monitoring is essential in the first hour after administration of the spinal injection. Clinical studies are awaited to confirm that such a refined epidural technique results in an improved obstetric outcome.

ROPIVACAINE (NAROPIN)

This is a long-acting amide-type local anaesthetic with a structure similar to that of bupivacaine, but giving greater separation of sensory and motor blockade than bupivacaine. Animal studies have also shown that ropivacaine is less toxic than bupivacaine. It has been evaluated in comparison with bupivacaine for continuous epidural analgesia in labour, and it was found that the duration of motor block was significantly shorter in the group receiving ropivacaine.

Chapter FIVE

Normal Labour

CONDUCT OF THE SECOND STAGE

The position assumed by most women during the second stage of labour is the dorsal position, although it can also be managed with the mother in the left lateral position or in the sitting position on a birthing chair. The dorsal position is particularly helpful to the midwife, enabling her to support the perineum adequately when the head crowns, and also facilitates the performance of an episiotomy when the perineum becomes excessively stretched. To encourage her expulsive efforts, the parturient is instructed to pull on her thighs – a practice that helps her to concentrate on the perineum.

To avoid the occupational hazards of blood-borne diseases, particularly hepatitis B and retroviral infections, the midwife has to exercise caution as to the extent to which she can comply with the wishes of a patient who has planned to assume a particular position during the second stage of labour. The midwife should conduct the delivery in the position that allows her fullest control, whilst avoiding being splashed by blood and amniotic fluid.

At this stage, the midwife organizes her trolley after scrubbing her hands and donning a sterile gown and gloves. The trolley contains drapes, swabs, three bowls, two pairs of Spencer Wells artery forceps and two pairs of scissors.

Figures 5.1–5.20 illustrate the subsequent conduct of the second stage.

CONDUCT OF THE THIRD STAGE

In the active management of the third stage of labour, an injection of syntometrine (5 units of oxytocin and 0.5 mg of ergometrine) is given intramuscularly when the anterior shoulder is delivered. This has been shown to reduce postpartum blood loss significantly.

When the bulk of the placenta is delivered (**Figs 5.21–5.24**), it may help to twist the membranes – a manoeuvre that will strengthen the trailing membranes and gently aid their separation from the lower uterine segment.

After the delivery of the placenta, it is inspected to ensure its complete delivery with the membranes (**Fig. 5.25**).

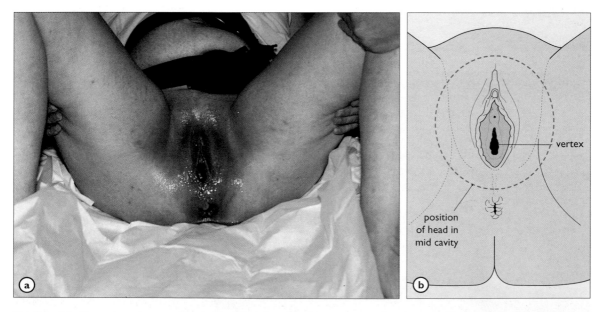

Fig. 5.1a & b The vertex appears at the vulva.

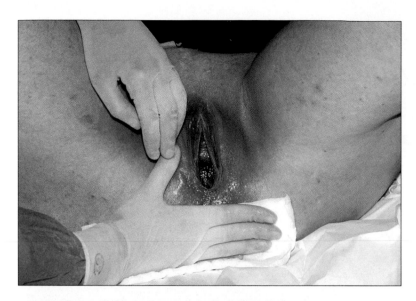

Fig. 5.2 As the parturient bears down during contractions, the perineum is supported with a gauze pad.

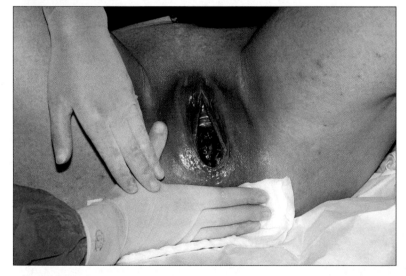

Fig. 5.3 With the advancement of the head, the introitus begins to appear to be thinned out, and the attendant prepares the perineum for episiotomy.

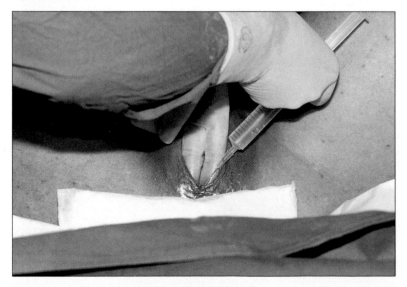

Figs 5.4–5.6 Lignocaine (5–10 ml of a 1% solution) is used to infiltrate the perineal skin and muscles, and the introitus and adjacent vaginal skin along the line of intended episiotomy.

Fig. 5.5

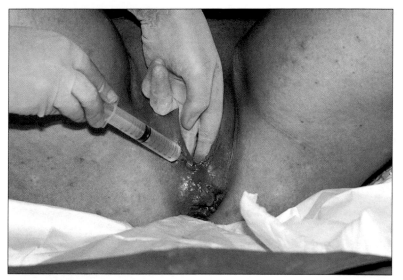

Fig. 5.6

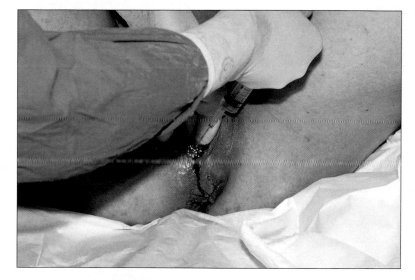

Fig. 5.7 The midwife waits for further descent of the fetal head, and for local anaesthesia to take effect, before performing the episiotomy.

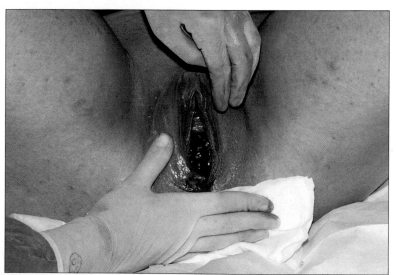

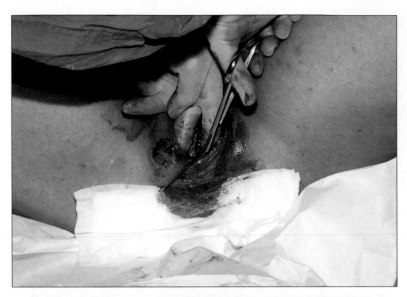

Fig. 5.8 The index and middle fingers of the left hand are inserted between the fetal head and the introitus, to raise the posterior vaginal wall and to allow the scissors blade to be inserted correctly under direct vision. A right posterolateral episiotomy is then performed; this is usually timed to coincide with the height of the uterine contraction. For left-handed attendants, there is no reason why the episiotomy should not be a left posterolateral incision.

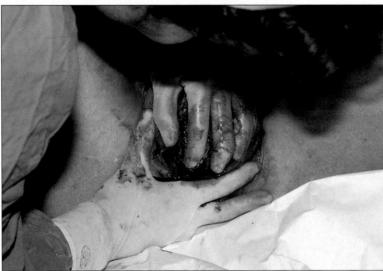

Figs 5.9 & 5.10 Further advancement of the head stretches the vulva, but the pressure on the surrounding tissue is reduced by the episiotomy. Thus the possibility of multiple vulvovaginal tears occurring is significantly reduced. The midwife guards the perineum with the right hand, and maintains head flexion with the left. This ensures that the smallest diameter of the head continues to be presented to the pelvic outlet.

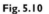

Fig. 5.10

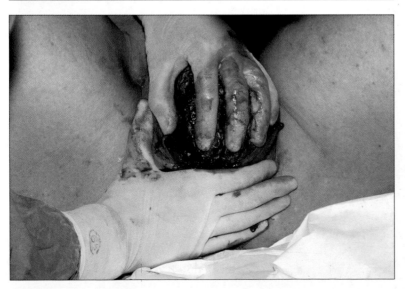

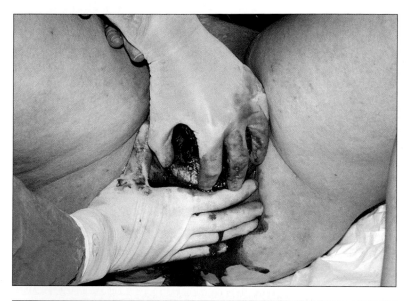

Fig. 5.11 The left hand releases the pressure on the head as the parietal eminences are born. Slight extension of the head is then encouraged, and the midwife continues to support the perineum and eases the face out of the introitus.

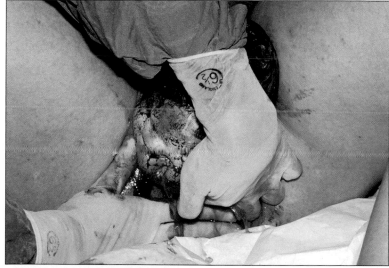

Figs 5.12 & 5.13 When the head is completely delivered, restitution follows immediately. The occiput is directed at 2 o'clock (45° rotation, clockwise), and the bisacromial diameter occupies the left oblique diameter of the inlet.

The midwife checks for any loop, or loops, of umbilical cord that may be twisted around the baby's neck. Should one or more such loops be found, they may be slipped over the baby's head. Alternatively, if the loops are found to be tight, one segment may be cut between clamps, and the cord untied, to avoid injury to it by the advancing baby.

Fig. 5.13

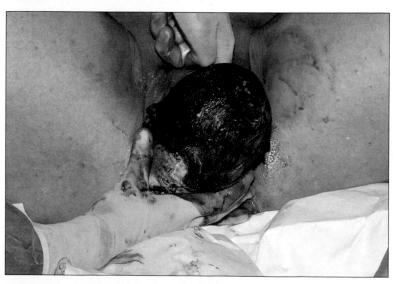

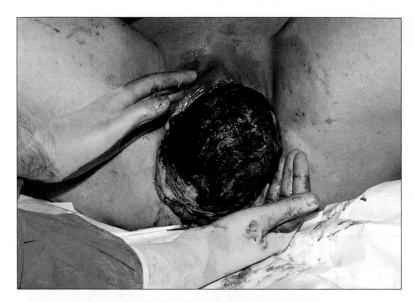

Fig. 5.14 External rotation of the head has just started. This is due to further descent, which results in the bisacromial diameter being aligned with the anteroposterior diameters of the lower pelvic cavity and outlet.

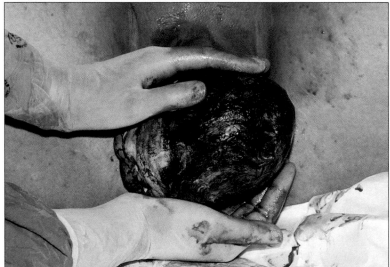

Fig. 5.15 External rotation has been completed (a further 45° rotation, clockwise).

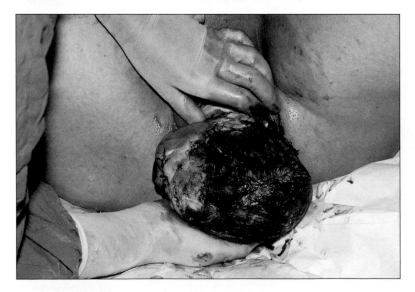

Fig. 5.16 With the onset of the subsequent contractions and after further descent, the anterior shoulder appears under the pubic symphysis.

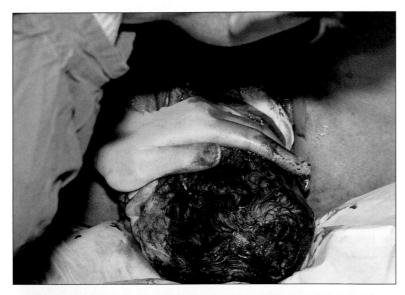

Figs 5.17–5.19 The baby's head is held by the midwife in the palms of both hands, and with a caudally directed pull, synchronized with maternal expulsive effort, the anterior shoulder is delivered, followed by the posterior.

Fig. 5.18

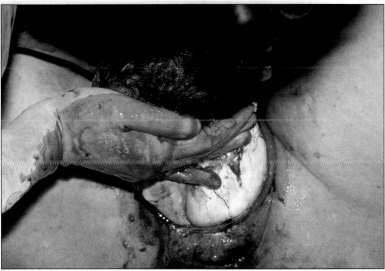

Fig. 5.19

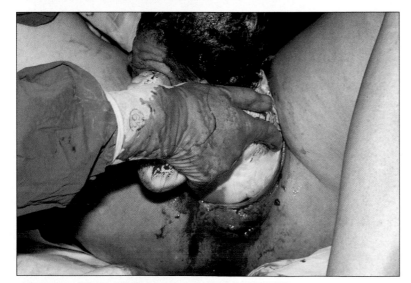

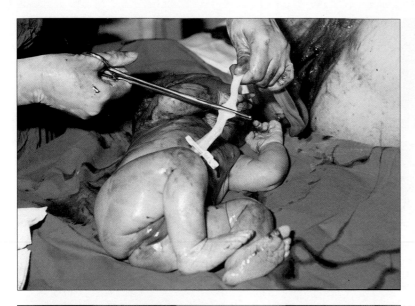

Fig. 5.20 After the delivery of the baby, the cord is clamped and cut.

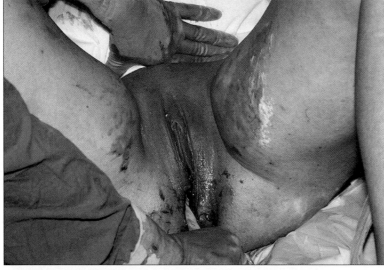

Fig. 5.21–5.24 In order to deliver the placenta, controlled cord traction is applied. The uterus is held posteriorly and cephalad with the left hand, and the umbilical cord pulled in a downward direction and caudad with the right. The reason for supporting the uterus is to prevent its inversion. As the placenta descends into the vagina, it is important to deliver it gently, lest the membranes be torn.

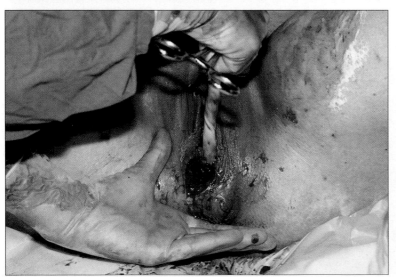

Fig. 5.22

Fig. 5.23

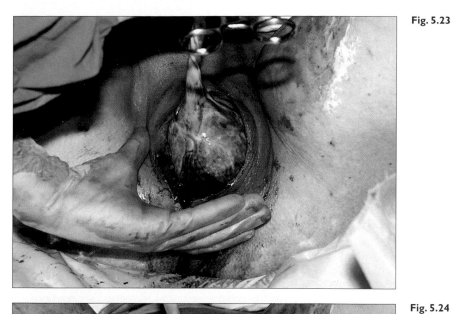

Fig. 5.24

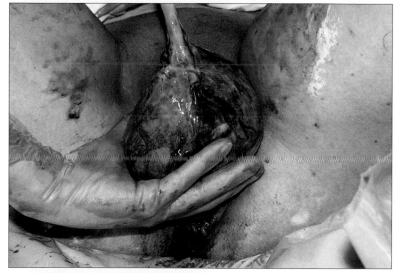

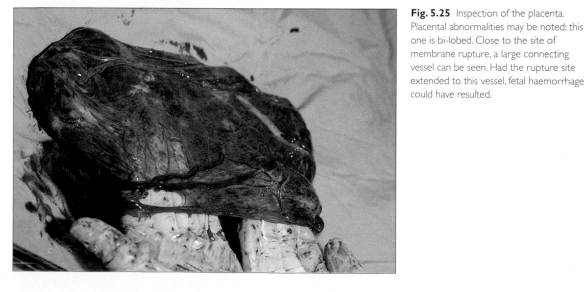

Fig. 5.25 Inspection of the placenta. Placental abnormalities may be noted; this one is bi-lobed. Close to the site of membrane rupture, a large connecting vessel can be seen. Had the rupture site extended to this vessel, fetal haemorrhage could have resulted.

SHOULDER DYSTOCIA

It is appropriate, at this juncture, to discuss a very serious complication, shoulder dystocia, that may occur during the second stage of labour in the delivery of macrosomic babies, especially those heavier than 4500 g. The incidence of shoulder dystocia varies between one and two cases per 1000 deliveries; it carries a perinatal and neonatal mortality rate of 20%, and in those babies who survive the risk of brachial palsy is 30%. The gravity of this condition stems from the fact that, in many instances, the labour initially progresses normally and is therefore attended by less experienced personnel than the condition demands. It is not until the fetal head is delivered that the potential problem becomes apparent. The cheeks clear the vulva very slowly, if at all, and restitution takes place, but external rotation occurs only rarely and very slowly. Attempts at vaginal examination are fruitless, as the entire birth canal is occupied by the fetal chest. However, the anterior shoulder may be felt just above the symphysis pubis.

On recognizing shoulder dystocia, the attendant must act very quickly, and summon the obstetrician immediately. Meanwhile, the patient is put in an exaggerated lithotomy position, a generous episiotomy is performed, and suprapubic pressure is applied by an assistant. These efforts, combined with the standard traction on the baby's head, may help to resolve this potential disaster. If delivery is not accomplished, it is not unreasonable – and is in fact a life-saving manoeuvre – to break one clavicle, thus compressing the bisacromial diameter; this is achieved by applying pressure with the thumb, on the anterior clavicle, against the pubic ramus. Fortunately, bone healing in the neonatal period is rapid, and residual disability is minimal.

There are manoeuvres described in various text books that involve rotating the baby's shoulder within the vagina, and attempting to deliver the posterior shoulder first from under the pubic symphysis. However, were there sufficient space to allow the introduction of the operator's hand, it would be possible to deliver the shoulder anyway! Furthermore, to apply these rotating manoeuvres in the absence of general anaesthesia or of an effective epidural block would entail the risk of causing neurogenic shock to the mother. Such manoeuvres are thus often ineffective, and the baby is usually dead by the time it is delivered.

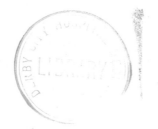

Chapter SIX

Resuscitation of the Newborn

Emergence into extrauterine life, with its attendant noises, temperature and tactile sensations, stimulates the onset of breathing. With the first few breaths after birth, the infant's lungs fill with air, displacing the lung fluid that was present during intrauterine life. During vaginal delivery, up to one-third of fetal lung fluid is expelled by thoracic compression; the remainder is rapidly absorbed into the pulmonary lymphatics and capillaries. Surfactant, usually produced in adequate quantities from 34 weeks' gestation, forms a monolayer lining the alveoli and reduces the work of breathing and prevents alveolar collapse in expiration. Clamping of the umbilical cord, inflation of the lungs with air and increases in pulmonary venous and systemic arterial oxygen saturation result in closure of the ductus arteriosus and increased blood flow through the lungs.

The overwhelming majority of babies born normally at term breathe immediately and do not require any resuscitation. Approximately 70% of babies needing resuscitation are born in situations in which the need for help can be anticipated and a paediatrician can be called to be present at the delivery. High-risk situations include preterm delivery, fetal distress, meconium staining of the liquor,

intrauterine growth retardation, multiple deliveries, Rhesus haemolytic disease and heavy maternal sedation or anaesthesia. Low forceps deliveries and elective caesarean sections at term are rarely followed by the need for resuscitation unless other risk factors co-exist. However, 30% of babies needing resuscitation are born with no prior warning of impending problems. It is therefore essential that anyone supervising a delivery should be skilled in basic neonatal life support and be able to start effective resuscitation whilst awaiting for the arrival of staff skilled in advanced resuscitation techniques.

The essential equipment for neonatal resuscitation consists of a shelf on which to place the baby, a supply of oxygen under pressure, a range of soft-edged face-masks (e.g. Laerdal), a T-piece connector, and a 30-cm H_2O pressure blow-off device (**Fig. 6.1**). Alternatively, the face-masks may be used with a self-inflating bag (preferably 400 ml volume) incorporating a 30-cm H_2O blow-off valve and a rebreathing reservoir, for example Laerdal (**Fig. 6.2**) or Ambubag. Useful additional equipment includes a stethoscope, suction apparatus and a range of suction catheters, endotracheal tubes (sizes 2.5, 3.0 and 3.5 mm i.d.), a laryngoscope fitted

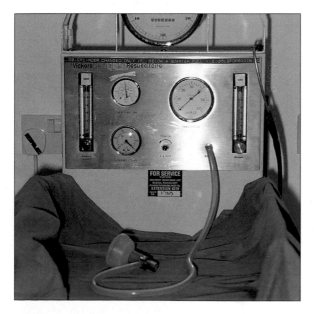

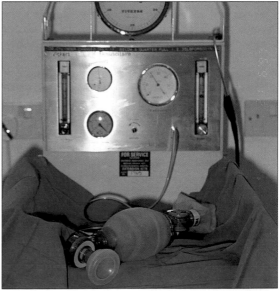

Fig. 6.1 Close-up of resuscitation platform with tubing, T-piece and mask.

Fig. 6.2 Close-up of resuscitation platform with 400-ml bag, reservoir bag and mask.

with a straight blade (e.g. Oxford pattern) and a supply of umbilical catheters. Neonatal resuscitation in hospitals is usually performed on a resuscitaire (**Fig. 6.3**), which provides, in addition, a firm surface, lighting, a radiant heat source to keep the baby warm and a clock with which to time events during the resuscitation.

The most important 'drug' for use during neonatal resuscitation is oxygen. Other drugs are rarely needed, and only a very limited range need be stocked on the resuscitaire. They should include adrenaline (1:10 000), 10% dextrose in water and 0.9% sodium chloride. Naloxone (Narcan) is useful for reversing the effect of pethidine given to the mother during labour, but it is not a resuscitation drug. Calcium has not been proven to have a role in neonatal resuscitation, and need not be stocked.

Resuscitaires and their attendant equipment should be in full working order and the drug tray should be fully stocked at all times. It should be the responsibility of the midwife conducting the delivery to check the equipment, correct any deficiencies and turn on the overhead heater before the baby is born.

Assessment of the need for resuscitation begins at the moment the baby is fully expelled from the birth canal, when the clock on the resuscitaire should be started. Babies who immediately begin crying and turn pink need only to be dried with a warm towel and then handed to their mother to be cuddled. Babies who do not breathe immediately should be transferred to the resuscitaire wrapped in a warm, dry towel and be placed on the platform beneath the radiant heater. It is essential to keep the baby warm (**Fig. 6.4**). The baby should then be evaluated for airway, breathing and circulation.

The airway should be opened by deflexing the neck to a neutral, not extended, position, and the mouth and nose should be gently suctioned to remove blood and fluid. The suction catheter should not be passed blindly to the back of the throat, because to do so may cause apnoea and bradycardia. The baby should then be evaluated for breathing by watching for chest movements and listening and feeling for airflow through the nose. The circulation is assessed by counting the pulse rate at the brachial artery and listening to the heart with a stethoscope. Normal newborn babies have heart rates faster than 100 beats/min. If the heart rate is 80 beats/min or slower, then immediate ventilation and cardiac massage are required.

A long-established method of recording the baby's condition at birth is the Apgar score, which documents Appearance, Pulse rate, Grimace in response to nasal suction, Activity and Respiratory effort (**Fig. 6.5**). However, the Apgar score is rarely calculated accurately at the time of resuscitation, and it is more informative to record the baby's condition in words that describe the respiratory effort and pulse rate.

Babies with a patent airway and effective ventilation who are slow to turn pink will benefit from oxygen delivered to the face by face-mask. Care should be taken to avoid chilling the baby with an indiscriminate blast of cold oxygen

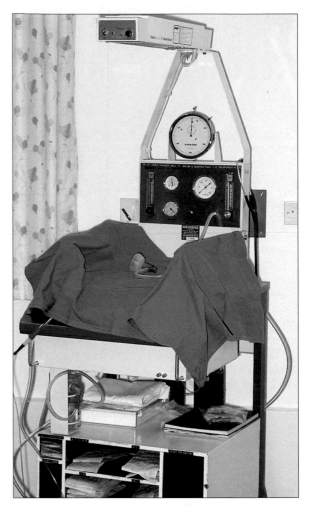

Fig. 6.3 The resuscitaire.

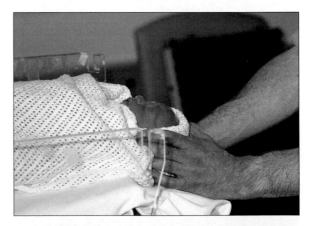

Fig. 6.4 The baby must not be allowed to get cold. Once placed on the resuscitaire, the baby should be dried to reduce heat loss by evaporation. The wet towel should then be removed and replaced with a warm, dry one. The baby's heart rate, respiration, colour and tone should then be assessed.

The Apgar scoring system

Signs

Score	Appearance (colour)	Pulse rate	Grimace (response to nasal suction)	Activity (muscle tone)	Respiratory effort
0	Blue, pale	Absent	No response	Floppy	Absent
1	Body pink, extremities blue	Less than 100 beats/min	Grimace	Some flexion of extremities	Slow, irregular
2	Completely pink	Greater than 100 beats/min	Cough or sneeze	Active movements	Good, crying

Fig. 6.5 The Apgar scoring system. The Apgar score is calculated by scoring each of the five components and adding the scores to obtain the total score. This is conventionally performed 1 and 5 minutes after birth. The 1 minute score reflects the condition of the baby at birth and, if low, indicates the need for resuscitation. The 5-minute score reflects the initial response to resuscitation, and is of greater long-term prognostic significance.

across the face and chest. If the baby is not breathing, then assisted ventilation should be commenced immediately.

Assisted ventilation should begin via a face-mask tightly applied over the baby's nose and mouth to obtain a good seal and connected to either a T-connector, 30-cm H_2O pressure blow-off valve and pressurized oxygen supply (**Fig. 6.6**), or a 400-ml self-inflating bag with a built-in blow-off valve connected to the oxygen supply and fitted with a rebreathing reservoir (**Fig. 6.7**). In the former case, inflation of the lungs is achieved by occluding the open end of the T-piece; in the latter, it is produced by squeezing the bag. In both cases, the first few

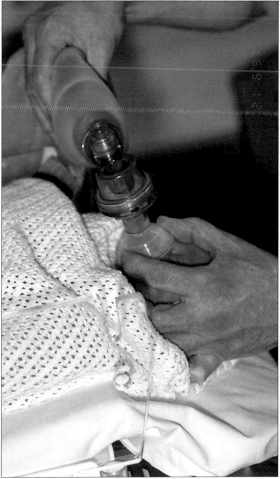

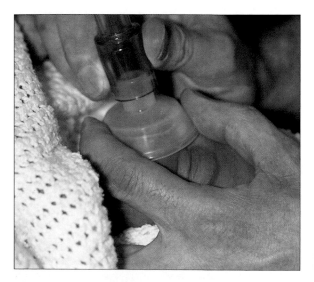

Fig. 6.6 Face-mask and T-piece applied to the baby's face.

Fig. 6.7 Face-mask and self-inflating bag applied to the baby's face.

breaths should last approximately 2 seconds, in order to inflate the lungs with air and displace lung fluid. Subsequent inflations should be shorter. The operator should watch for chest movement, to ensure that the technique is being performed effectively.

Many babies needing assisted ventilation respond very quickly, with acceleration of the heart rate and the onset of regular breathing. If the baby does not respond promptly, paediatric assistance should be urgently summoned, as intubation of the trachea (**Fig. 6.8**), vascular access and adrenaline may be needed. If the heart rate is 80 beats/min or less despite effective face-mask ventilation, then cardiac massage should be commenced, whilst ventilation is continued.

Cardiac massage should be performed by placing the tips of two fingers on the sternum in the midline one finger's breadth below an imaginary line joining the two nipples (**Fig. 6.9**). The sternum should be depressed to a depth equal to approximately half the anteroposterior diameter of the chest,

and allowed to spring back. Massage should be performed at a rate of 100 compressions per minute until the heart rate is greater than 100 beats/min. If two operators are available, then one can continue ventilation whilst the other performs cardiac massage, by encircling the baby's chest with both hands with the fingers behind the baby's back and the thumbs one on top of the other, in the position described above (**Fig. 6.10**). The technique of external cardiac massage may be more effective than the 'two finger' technique.

When the baby is breathing satisfactorily and the heart rate is greater than 100 beats/min, the baby can be given to the mother to be cuddled and a decision made as to where the baby should be nursed after leaving the delivery room. Term babies who have responded quickly to resuscitation and are well should go to the postnatal ward with their mothers. Other babies may need to be admitted to a Neonatal Intensive Care Unit or Transitional Care Ward for further care.

Fig. 6.8 Intubation.

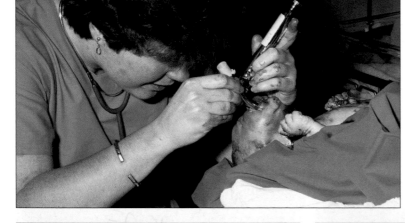

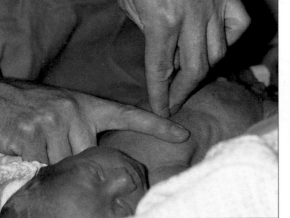

Fig. 6.9 Cardiac massage using two fingers.

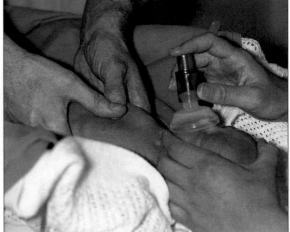

Fig. 6.10 Cardiac massage using thumbs, with fingers encircling the baby's trunk.

Chapter SEVEN

Common Problems Immediately After Delivery

EPISIOTOMY REPAIR

An episiotomy involves a small surgical incision made into the perineum in order to avoid excessive distension of the vaginal tissues, the perineal muscles and the vulva; it is performed in order that a ragged perineal or vaginal tear is avoided in favour of a clean-edged incision that is more likely to be repaired satisfactorily. It also helps to reduce the resistance against the advancing presenting part. The episiotomy can be performed in three positions – median, posterolateral and mediolateral – each serving the same purpose, but differing in their manifestation of the complications and sequelae to be taken into consideration, namely:

- extent of blood loss
- ease of repair
- degree of pain
- incidence of dyspareunia
- risk of injury to the wall of the rectum

The technique of perineal repair is based on three basic surgical principles:

- Identification of the structures involved.
- Assurance that a dead space is not left.
- Careful apposition of the anatomical layers.

It is important to note that the medial side of the vaginal component of episiotomy is always longer than the lateral side, because the episiotomy cuts into a 'cylinder', the side of which is still attached to the pelvic side-wall, while the medial portion hangs down without attachment (see **Fig. 3.10**). In episiotomy repair, except that of midline episiotomy, the needle must therefore bite a slightly longer edge on the medial side than on the lateral. This helps to achieve a good apposition of the vaginal edges, the hymenal ring and the fourchette.

REPAIR OF MIDLINE EPISIOTOMY
(Figs 7.1–7.5)

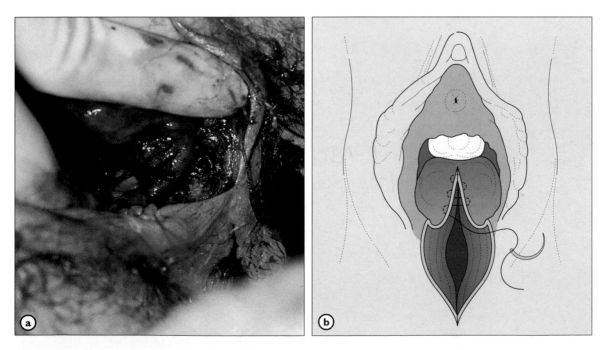

Fig. 7.1a & b After the infiltration of 10 ml of local anaesthetic (10% lignocaine) into the perineal skin and lower-third of the vagina, a tampon is inserted in the vagina to prevent blood obscuring the field of suturing. The first step is to secure the apex of the vaginal wound.

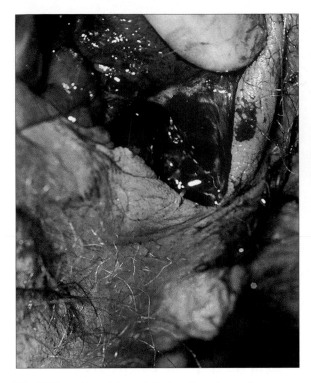

Fig. 7.2 Apposition of the vaginal edges through a continuous suture. Note the edges of the introitus.

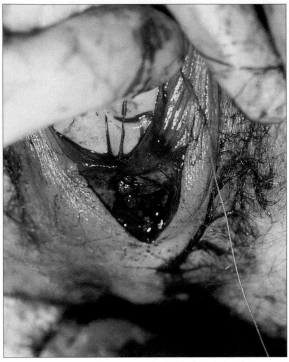

Fig. 7.3 The suture is buried under the the vaginal skin, and muscular structures of the perineal body are approximated.

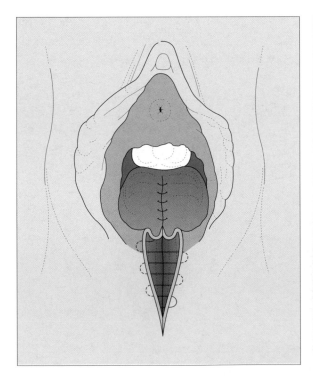

Fig. 7.4 When suturing of the perineal body has been completed, the stitch is continued in a subcuticular fashion, to repair the perineal skin.

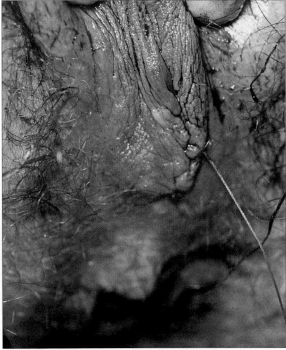

Fig. 7.5 The perineal skin is completely approximated.

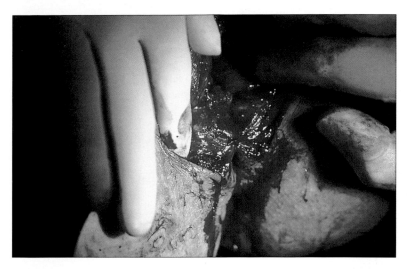

Fig. 7.6 Third-degree vaginal tear complicating midline episiotomy due to inadequately controlled delivery of the head.

REPAIR OF POSTEROLATERAL EPISIOTOMY
(Figs 7.7–7.18)

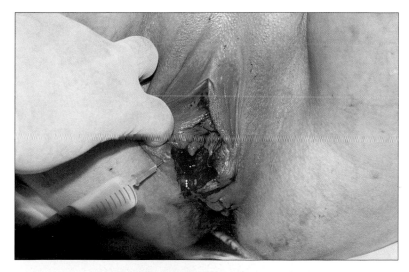

Figs 7.7 & 7.8 If the effects of the local anaesthetic given at the time of episiotomy have worn off, the perineal skin edges and the lower one-third of the vagina, on both sides of the episiotomy, are infiltrated with 1% lignocaine. It is important to allow 5 minutes for an effective block to be achieved.

The suture material commonly used is chromic cat-gut, although better results can be achieved with polyglactin sutures (Vicryl).

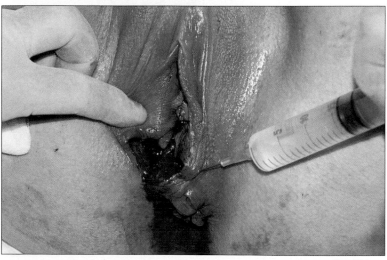

Fig. 7.8

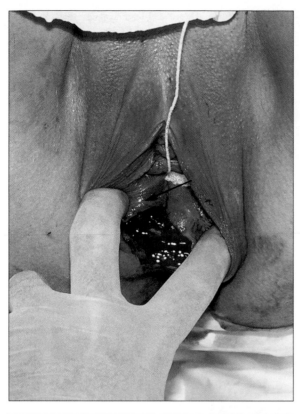

Figs 7.9 & 7.10 When episiotomy repair is undertaken, a tampon is inserted to prevent uterine blood loss from obscuring the operative field. The first step is to identify the apex (arrow) of the vaginal component of the episiotomy, which is secured by a stitch.

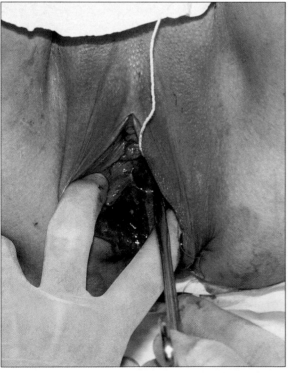

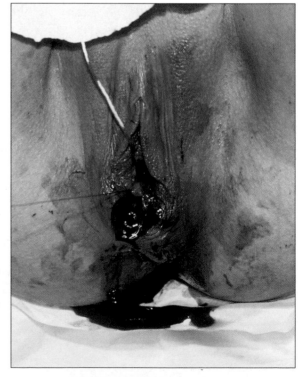

Fig. 7.10

Fig. 7.11 Continuous suturing is then performed to close the vagina, until the edges of the hymenal ring are approximated, with careful apposition.

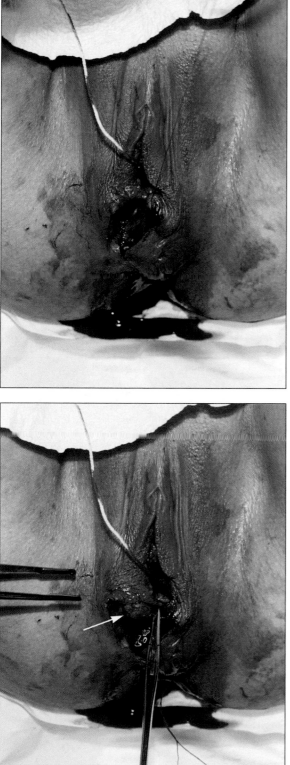

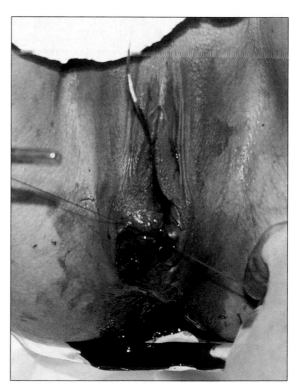

Fig. 7.12 Two or three more bites are required outside the hymenal ring, to appose the posterior ends of the cut fourchette and labia majora.

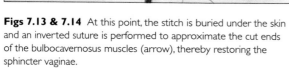

Figs 7.13 & 7.14 At this point, the stitch is buried under the skin and an inverted suture is performed to approximate the cut ends of the bulbocavernosus muscles (arrow), thereby restoring the sphincter vaginae.

Fig. 7.14

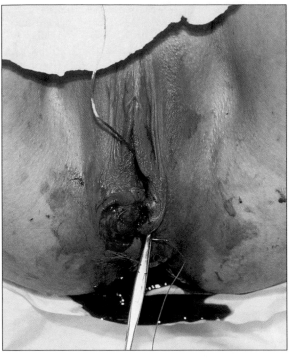

Figs 7.15 & 7.16 Two to four interrupted sutures are applied, to bring together the deep muscles of the perineum and the cut edges of the levator ani muscle.

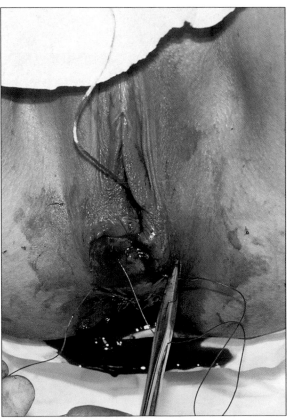

Fig. 7.16

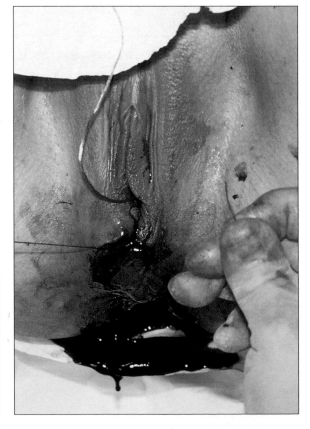

Fig. 7.17 Another layer of inverted, interrupted sutures is required to approximate the superficial muscles of the perineum.

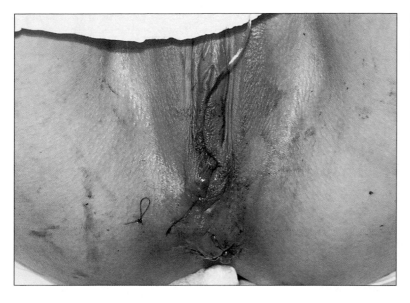

Fig. 7.18 The fourth layer of episiotomy repair is that of the perineal skin; repair can be achieved by means of subcuticular or interrupted sutures.

REPAIR OF MEDIOLATERAL EPISIOTOMY
(Figs 7.19–7.32)

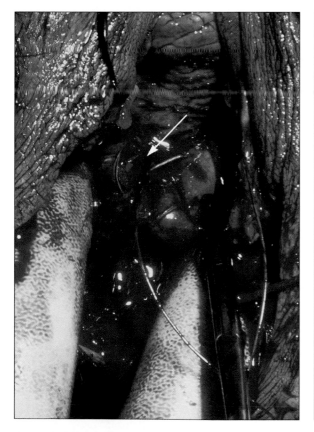

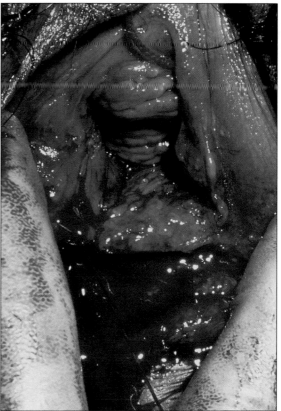

Figs 7.19 & 7.20 In mediolateral episiotomy, the initial steps taken to repair posterolateral episiotomy are similarly followed; the vaginal skin is approximated by means of a continuous chromic cat-gut suture, after the apex of the vaginal wound (arrow) has been secured.

Fig. 7.20

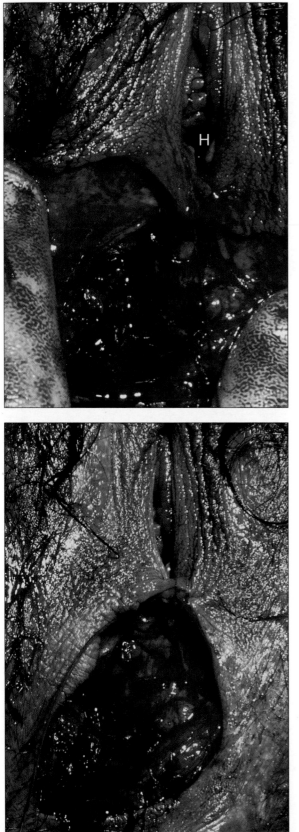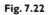

Figs 7.21 & 7.22 When the continuous vaginal suture reaches the hymenal ring (H), it is advanced further until the posterior ends of the fourchette and labia majora are approximated.

Fig. 7.22

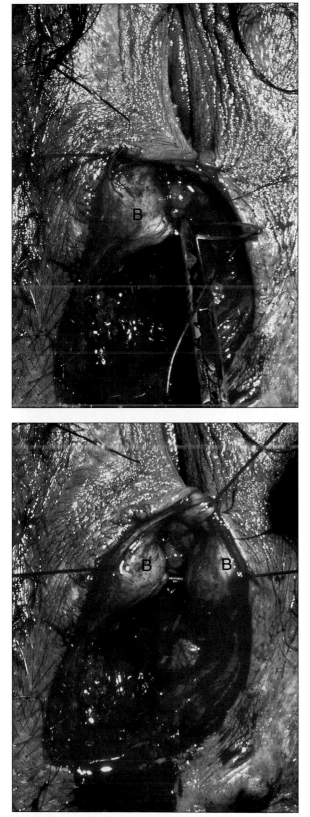

Figs 7.23–7.25 The suture is buried under the skin, and both edges of the cut sphincter vaginae (the cut edges of the bulbocavernosus muscles, B) are brought together.

Fig. 7.24

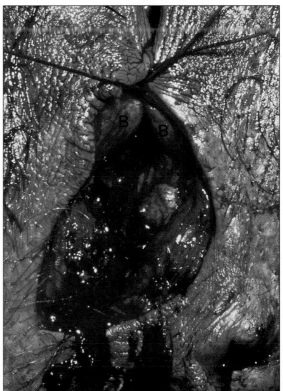

Fig. 7.25

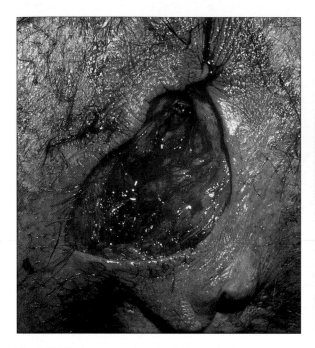

Fig. 7.26 The deep perineal muscles, including the levator ani, are approximated with interrupted sutures.

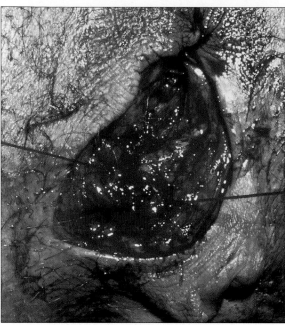

Fig. 7.27 A small, but active, bleeding point has been identified lateral to the inferior anal sphincter, and is secured separately.

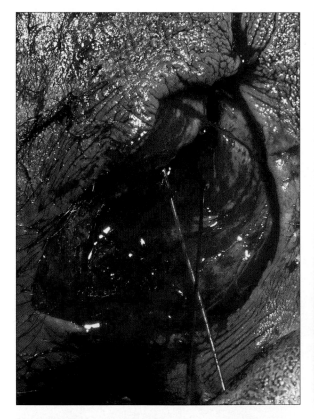

Figs 7.28 & 7.29 The deep muscles of the perineum are approximated with inverted interrupted sutures, using chromic cat-gut.

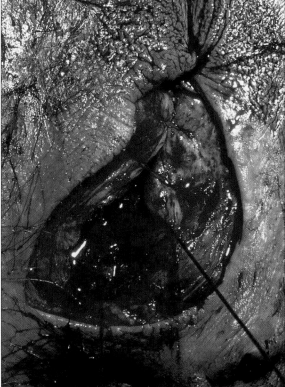

Fig. 7.29

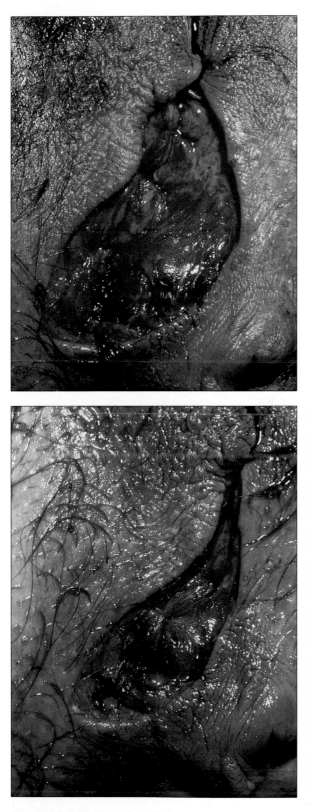

Fig. 7.30 A layer of inverted interrupted sutures of the same material is then applied, to bring together the superficial perineal muscles.

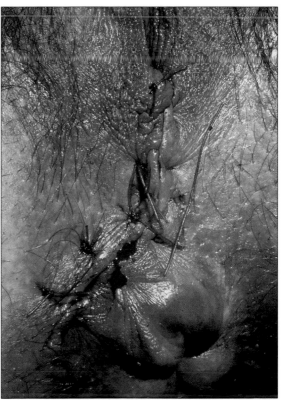

Figs 7.31 & 7.32 The perineal skin is approximated with interrupted mattress sutures, using chromic cat-gut (although the use of Vicryl sutures would give better results).

Fig. 7.32

VAGINAL TEARS

Before the different types and modes of repair of these injuries are described, it is important to note the following:

- The surgical principles of the repair are the same as for the repair of an episiotomy.
- The vagina and the cervix should be carefully inspected and the identification of an obvious bleeder in any tear should not preclude the conduct of a careful and thorough examination of the rest of the genital tract. Vaginal tears might not extend to the perineum, and therefore might not be obvious from the outside. Similarly, these tears may involve only a small part of the rectal mucosa. Less vigilant evaluation may result in vulval haematoma, or vesical or rectal fistulae.
- These tears are very painful to touch and adequate anaesthesia must be ensured; sometimes the patient may even require a general anaesthetic.

Perineal tears are classified as first-, second- or third-degree tears.

First-Degree Perineal Tears. These involve the perineal, vulval or vaginal skin, leaving the underlying tissues visibly intact. On occasion, such injuries may involve a small but significant bleeder, and consequently require a suture or two to stop the bleeding. Sometimes the injury involves the periurethral area, but unless a bleeder is found, there is no need for suturing. Infrequently, when a periurethral

tear has occurred, the patient may require an indwelling catheter to relieve urinary retention, secondary to severe dysuria. Labial tears may occur on one or both sides, but they heal well in most instances. If the tear has cut across the labia, reconstruction is warranted; a few subcuticular interrupted No. 3/0 Vicryl sutures may be all that is required. Care and meticulousness give excellent long-term results.

Second-Degree Perineal Tears. In addition to the skin injuries described above, second-degree perineal tears involve injuries to the superficial and deep muscles of the perineum part of the levator ani muscle, including the anal sphincters. The principles laid down for episiotomy repair, with particular attention to anatomical apposition, help a great deal in the management of what can be very difficult conditions. Repair of the anal sphincters, if they are involved, must be performed independently of other perineal muscle repair, using interrupted Vicryl sutures.

A poorly judged episiotomy may extend and become an irregular, profusely bleeding tear. In the example shown in **Figs 7.33–7.44**, the attendant gave the patient an inadequate episiotomy, which resulted in an extended second-degree perineal tear.

REPAIR OF SECOND-DEGREE PERINEAL TEARS
(**Figs 7.33–7.44**)

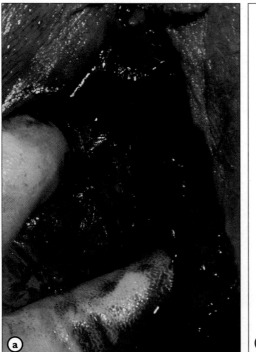

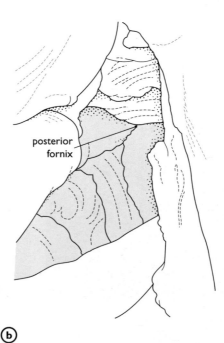

Figs 7.33 & 7.34
The skin of the lateral vaginal wall is split up to the posterior fornix (**Fig. 7.33a & b**) and the apex has been secured (**Fig. 7.34**).

posterior fornix

Fig. 7.34

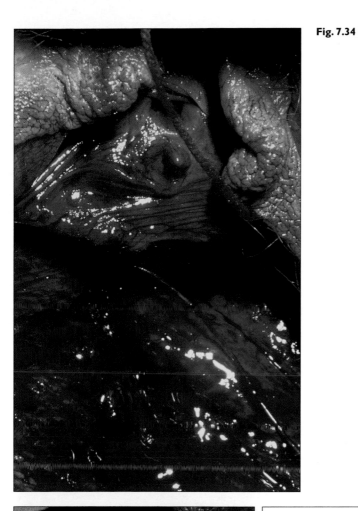

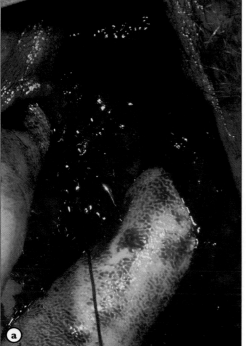

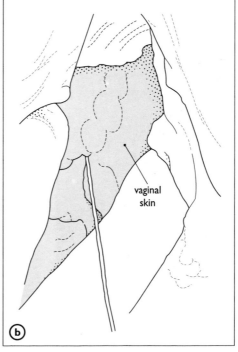

vaginal skin

Figs 7.35 & 7.36
Continuous suturing of the vaginal skin is performed (**Fig. 7.35a & b**), until the hymenal ring is reached (**Fig. 7.36**).

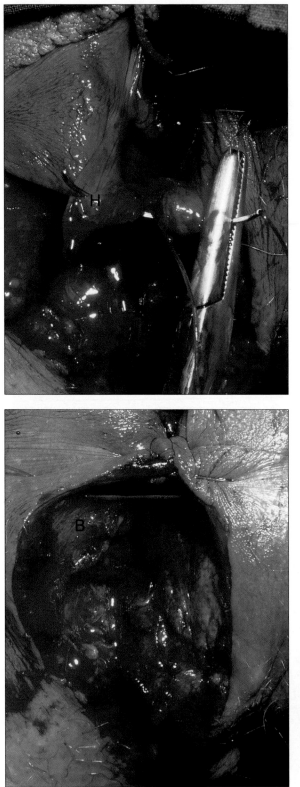

Fig. 7.36 The hymenal ring (H) is reached.

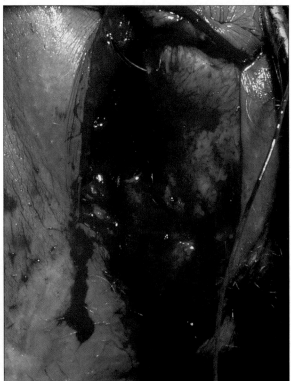

Figs 7.37–7.39 The bulbocavernosus muscle (B) on each side is approximated, so that the sphincter vaginae is refashioned.

Fig. 7.38

Fig. 7.39

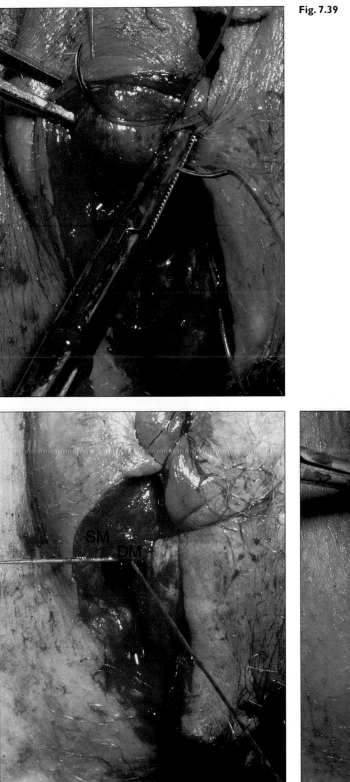

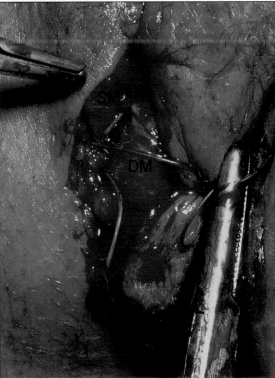

Fig. 7.40 The deep perineal muscles (DM) are then approximated with interrupted sutures.

Fig. 7.41 Likewise, the superficial perineal muscles (SM) are approximated.

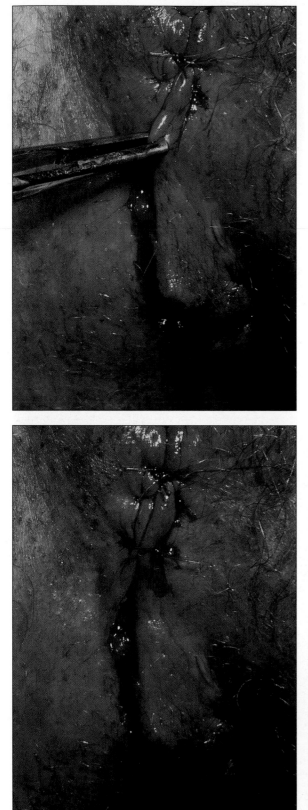

Figs 7.42–7.44 The perineal skin is secured with interrupted sutures. Note the extension of the tear into the anal skin.

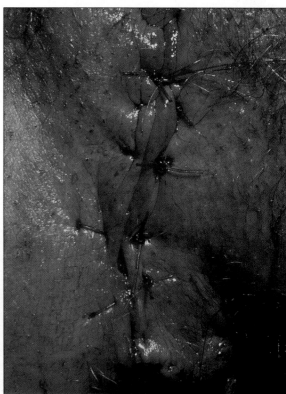

Fig. 7.43

Fig. 7.44

Third-Degree Perineal Tears (*see *Fig. 7.6). This term is generally used to describe a breach of the rectal mucosa, although some authors classify an injury to the anal sphincter as a third-degree perineal tear and one to the rectal mucosa as a fourth-degree perineal tear. The provision of adequate pain relief is essential, so that all tissue planes are identified and the extent of injury carefully ascertained. The fundamental part of the repair is to apply interrupted plain cat-gut sutures, inverting the mucosal edges into the gut lumen. The muscularis layer is carefully sutured with interrupted No. 3/0 Vicryl. The remainder of the perineal tear is repaired as above.

MANUAL REMOVAL OF THE PLACENTA

This forms part of the management of a lengthy third stage of labour in which one of the following may be a complicating factor:

* the placenta is morbidly adherent
* there is significant haemorrhage
* the uterus is flaccid and has failed to retract

The wide use of epidural anaesthesia has encouraged many practitioners to procure the retained placenta without recourse to general anaesthesia. General anaesthesia, aiming at uterine muscle relaxation, offers a pragmatic approach in difficult cases, particularly when a constriction ring in the lower uterine segment has developed.

Technique

The operator's hand is introduced into the uterus and, having located the placenta, the fingers are directed towards its lower edge. With one hand on the abdomen supporting the uterus, the fingers of the other hand search for a separation plane at the lower edge of the placenta. Steady movement of the fingers behind the placenta, sidewards and cephalad, will ultimately separate the placenta, which is delivered in one piece (**Fig. 7.45**).

Current concerns about blood-borne diseases such as hepatitis B and HIV have led to the development of protective measures against contamination of the operator from potentially infected patient's blood. Such measures are all the more necessary during intrauterine manipulations in which blood will inevitably trickle down the operator's elbow. The author's opinion is that adequate protection is derived by wearing arm-length gloves that are attached to the shoulder with adhesive tape, beneath a standard gown and with standard latex gloves over them. Impervious gowns may be a better option, but they are expensive.

When the placenta has been procured, digital exploration ensures that the uterus is indeed empty, and then its firmness is also assessed. In order to ensure that the uterus is adequately contracted, ecbolic drugs such as oxytocin, ergometrine or prostaglandin F2α may be administered; otherwise, the uterus may haemorrhage and on occasion an acute uterine inversion may ensue.

POSTPARTUM HAEMORRHAGE

The management of postpartum haemorrhage must include attention to the following factors:

* Induction of uterine contraction by abdominal 'massage' or by bimanual compression until the ecbolic agents begin to work.
* Whether the placenta and membranes have been completely delivered.
* Provision of adequate intravenous infusion.
* A check on coagulation mechanisms.
* The need for blood transfusion.

If these measures do not succeed in stopping the bleeding, it is important to examine the uterus for any retained placental tissue or membranes. In undertaking such an examination, one must not ignore the possibility of bleeding due to cervical or vaginal tears, and a careful examination of the lower genital tract should therefore be performed. In these cases, general anaesthesia is required.

PRIMARY POSTPARTUM HAEMORRHAGE

Primary postpartum haemorrhage is defined as blood loss *per vaginam* in excess of 500 ml during the first 24 hours after the delivery of the baby. The most common causes are uterine atony and lacerations of the lower genital tract. Other causes include morbid adhesion of the placenta, total or partial placenta accreta, coagulation defects and uterine inversion.

Because of the high vascularity of the reproductive organs during pregnancy, a large amount of blood may be lost in a short time. When confronted with this situation, one must first ensure that the placenta has been delivered and is complete, and establish whether the mother has received syntometrine. It is important to ensure that the bladder is empty. The obstetrician places his hand on the abdomen and rubs the uterus to produce a contraction; if uterine atony persists, bimanual compression is exerted on the uterus (**Fig. 7.46**).

The bimanual compression is performed by the obstetrician placing a fist in the anterior fornix to push against the anterior uterine wall, with the other hand pressing against the posterior uterine wall *per abdomen*. During this time, an intravenous cannula should be established and blood samples drawn for cross-matching. Ergometrine is given, together with an infusion of oxytocin. If this fails to produce uterine contraction, an injection of prostaglandin F2α (Haemabate) given into the myometrium is usually effective. During resuscitation, it is vital to avoid prolonged hypotension as a result of hypovolaemia, as it may cause renal tubular necrosis or avascular necrosis of the anterior pituitary gland.

Continued bleeding at this stage indicates the need to explore the uterus for retained placental tissue, either manually or, if that is not possible, with a large blunt curette. The exploration, which is made with the patient under general anaesthesia, should also seek to identify a possible uterine rupture. The cervix and the vagina are also inspected for evidence of lacerations or haematoma formation (**Fig. 7.47**).

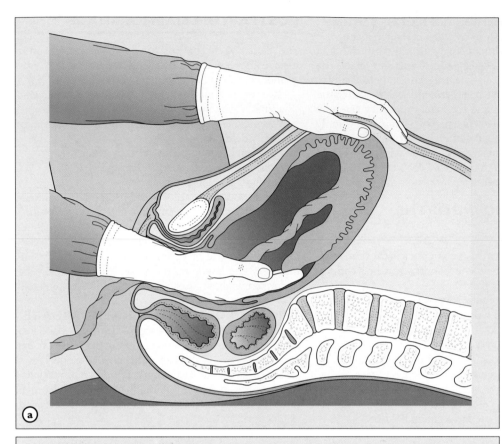

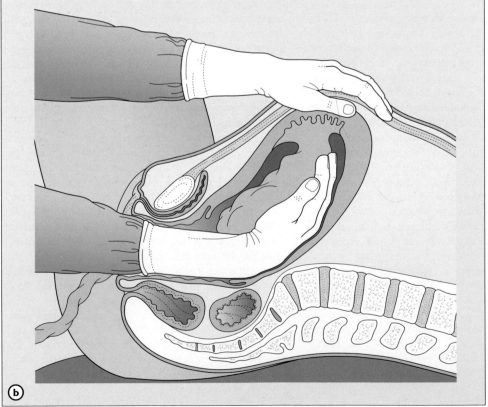

Fig. 7.45a & b
Manual removal of the placenta: the operator's hand is introduced into the uterus and the fingers, after locating the placenta, are directed towards its lower edge. The uterus is supported *per abdomen* with one hand, whilst the fingers of the other hand, at the lower edge of the placenta, search to find a separation plane (**a**). Steady movement of the fingers from side to side and cephalad, behind the placenta, will ultimately separate it from the uterus (**b**); the placenta is then delivered in one piece.

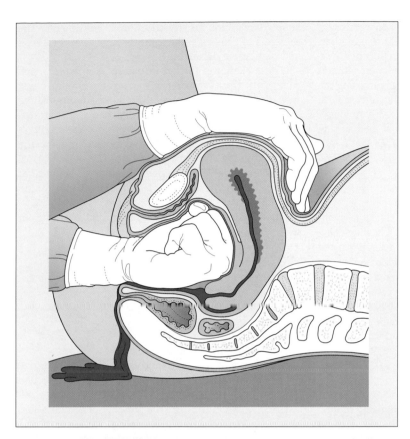

Fig. 7.46 Bimanual compression of the uterus.

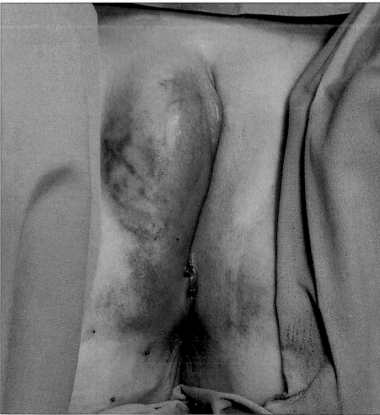

Fig. 7.47 Vulvar and paravaginal haematoma may develop rapidly following delivery and severe pain must alert the attendant. A fluctuant mass may appear at the vulva with discoloration of the overlying skin. Where the bleeding escapes into the paravaginal tissues a large collection of blood may develop unhindered under the pelvic peritoneum. Surgical treatment with evacuation of blood clots and securing the blood vessel(s) may suffice. The cavity created by the haematoma may be obliterated with mattress sutures. After incision of the haematoma and evacuation of clots no site of bleeding can be identified, in which case the vagina is packed firmly with a large gauze pack for 24 hours. In these cases an indwelling urinary catheter is required.

If postpartum haemorrhage continues, and when coagulation defects are excluded, laparotomy is indicated. In cases of rupture of the uterus, repair or subtotal hysterectomy may be required. In patients whose condition is stable, however, an attempt can be made to ligate the uterine artery or the anterior division of the internal iliac artery, to preserve the uterus. Alternatively, if an angiography service is available, embolization of the bleeding vessel may stall the bleeding (**Figs 7.48 & 7.49**). Postoperative antibiotic cover should be given for 5 days.

SECONDARY POSTPARTUM HAEMORRHAGE

Secondary postpartum haemorrhage is defined as haemorrhage occurring after the first 24 hours following delivery and up to 6 weeks postpartum. It is usually associated with retained placental tissue and the development of secondary infection, but retention of placental tissue is very rare after 4 weeks. Management involves careful history-taking, recording of vital signs, and abdominal and pelvic assessment to exclude the presence of parametrial induration or abscess formation. An ultrasound scan may be helpful in assessing the size of the uterus, and its contents; a characteristic of retained placental tissue is delayed involution of the uterus.

Vaginal swabs are obtained for bacteriological assessment, followed by antibiotic therapy comprising cephradine and metronidazole, which should be maintained for 7 days. Evacuation of the uterus is undertaken, and any material recovered is also sent for bacteriological assessment.

AMNIOTIC FLUID EMBOLISM

Amniotic fluid embolism is an extremely dangerous and almost untreatable condition in obstetrics; recorded incidences ranging from 1 in 4000 to 1 in 80 000 pregnancies, and it is responsible for 4–10% of maternal deaths. Amniotic fluid embolism also leads to disseminated intravascular coagulation, which is then responsible for the death of 40% of those surviving the acute embolic event. Amniotic fluid embolism may complicate:

- termination of pregnancy in its various forms
- placental abruption
- tumultuous labour
- delivery of a macrosomic fetus
- caesarean section
- uterine rupture

A consequence of the disruption of the anatomical relationship between the chorioamniotic membrane, placenta and uterine wall is the disruption of the integrity of the uterine vasculature; hence, amniotic fluid gains access to the mother's systematic circulation. The amniotic fluid elements lodge in the pulmonary microcirculation, where their presence seems to induce a transient increase in pulmonary artery pressure as a result of anaphylactic-like vasoconstriction in response to the presence of prostaglandins, meconium, vernix caseosa and particulate debris.

These elements further initiate a complement cascade, with the C5a component promoting leucocyte migration and aggregation within the vasculature. These effects in turn release inflammatory mediators that disrupt the capillary endothelium and alveolar architecture, leading to exudation of intravascular fluid into the interstitium and interalveolar space. The net effects of these events are severe hypoxia, leading to acute right ventricular failure and reduced cardiac output (acute cor pulmonale).

The condition manifests itself suddenly and, without warning, the patient develops:

- dyspnoea
- coughing, with pink frothy sputum
- cyanosis

These are followed by:

- apnoea
- loss of consciousness
- profound shock
- convulsions in 10–20% of cases

The diagnosis of amniotic fluid embolism can be established definitively only at autopsy, although antemortem diagnostic open-lung biopsy for those who survive the initial shock may demonstrate the presence of amniotic fluid debris. However, the main diagnostic technique used currently is cytological examination of maternal blood, in which positive staining for amniotic fluid debris confirms amniotic fluid embolism.

Management involves four major objectives:

1. *Effective ventilation.* In most cases sufficient oxygenation will be achieved by endotracheal intubation and mechanical ventilation with a volume-cycled respirator.
2. *Correction of shock.*
3. *Anticipation of disseminated intravascular coagulation.* Prepare cross-matched blood, fresh frozen plasma and platelets.
4. *Provision of supportive care.* Surveillance should focus especially on thermal instability, metabolic and electrolyte imbalances and, later on, the development of pulmonary infection.

UTERINE COMPLICATIONS

RUPTURE OF THE UTERUS

Rupture of the uterus may follow obstructed labour, dehiscence of caesarean section scar or the inappropriate use of oxytocic drugs. The clinical presentation is that of sudden abdominal pain, or of hypovolaemic shock. During labour, uterine contractions may cease or, if the placental circulation is compromised, the fetus may die. After the mother has been resuscitated, a laparotomy is performed and the extent of the damage is assessed. The uterus may be repaired in two layers, or a subtotal hysterectomy may be performed.

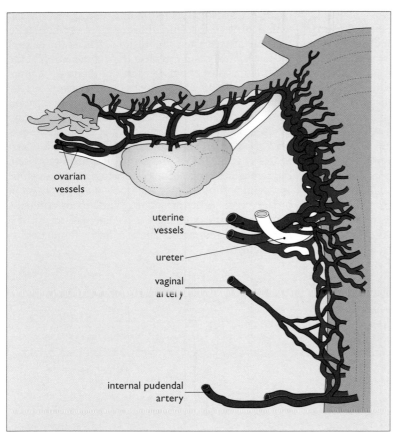

ovarian
vessels

uterine
vessels

ureter

vaginal
artery

internal pudendal
artery

Fig. 7.48 Blood supply to the pelvis and uterus: anatomical diagram.

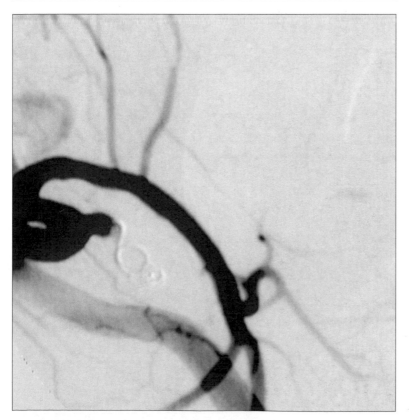

Fig. 7.49 Embolization coil introduced angiographically to block the anterior division of the internal iliac artery.

ACUTE UTERINE INVERSION

Strong traction on the umbilical cord of a fundally implanted placenta in the presence of uterine atony may result in the inversion of the uterus. The inversion may be complete, in which the fundus has advanced into the vagina and beyond, or partial, in which the fundus has not passed beyond the cervix. Morbid adherence of the placenta may be a factor, but only in a minority of cases. Uterine inversion is associated with profound shock, mainly as a result of haemorrhage.

The best treatment of a freshly inverted uterus is immediate reposition, followed by infusion of oxytocin. However, the condition is most commonly recognized when the patient is in a state of shock after delivery, in which case two adequate venous cannulae must be established to correct the shock, and the placenta must not be removed until the inversion is corrected. Repositioning of the uterus is conducted under general anaesthesia, with the use of tocolytic drugs or glyceryl trinitrate to relax the uterus. The manipulation starts at the edge of the inversion and aims to push the uterine wall past the constriction ring of muscle fibres of the lower uterine segment or the cervix. Incomplete uterine inversion may occur and may be diagnosed by abdominal palpation where a crater-like depression replaces the globular fundus. The management follows the same as that outlined above. Use of hydrodistension of the vagina, which results in stretching of the cervix, has been proposed, but sometimes it may be necessary to combine a vaginal approach with an abdominal one via a laparotomy in order to correct the inversion. When repositioning is complete, oxytocin infusion is commenced to ensure a firmly contracted uterus, and a course of antibiotics is also required.

Chapter EIGHT

Operative Vaginal Delivery

DECISION MAKING

To assess the suitability of any labour for operative vaginal delivery, the operator has to take into account the patient's antenatal record, her previous obstetric performance and whether the indication for intervention is maternal or fetal. From the mechanical point of view, the following must be observed to maximize the safety of the procedure:

1. *The pattern of cervimetric progress in labour.* If the rate of cervimetric progress is slower than 1 cm/hour, particularly in the second half of the first stage of labour, it may indicate inefficient uterine contractions, or reflect the presence of cephalopelvic disproportion, either absolute or relative, as a result of the fetal head lying in the occipitoposterior position. The operator must consider whether oxytocin has been used and for how long, if adequate anaesthesia is present, and whether there is evidence of fetal distress.

2. *Abdominal examination.* This is performed carefully, and enables the operator to define the fetal back and the proportion of the head that remains palpable *per abdomen*. The examination is sometimes difficult because of painful contractions, tender hypogastrium, the presence of a full bladder or a posterior position of the occiput.

3. *Vaginal examination.* Full dilatation of the cervix is confirmed first, particularly posteriorly, where a rim of cervix may be missed. An assessment of the adequacy of the pelvis in general and of the outlet is made, noting, for example, the convergence of the pubic rami, the prominence of the ischial spines and the forward curvature of the lower part of the sacrum and coccyx. The sacrum is palpated digitally to assess its concavity and whether the promontory of the sacrum is within reach. The greater sciatic notches are examined, to assess the capacity of the lower parts of the pelvic cavity. The fetal head is examined and the extent of caput formation and moulding are noted. The relation of the head to the ischial spines is also observed. The sagittal suture is palpated and its central position assessed, as asynclitism (parietal bone presentation) is said to be present when the sagittal suture deviates from the centre. Caput succedaneum may be advanced, making the identification of the fontanelles difficult; in these circumstances, a useful rule of thumb is that a palpable fontanelle is the anterior fontanelle. One must pay particular attention to the possibility of a soft tissue tumour occupying the pelvis, which may cause obstruction.

When the operator is satisfied that no contraindications exist to the undertaking of an operative vaginal delivery using the forceps or the ventouse (vacuum extraction), the operative instrument is applied to the fetal head, after which further checking is required. When first traction is applied, the extent of descent is assessed, and any difficulty encountered must alert the obstetrician to the possibility of malposition of the head, either in the form of the occipitoposterior position, or because of an unsuspected true pelvic contracture.

Most of the difficulties encountered during operative vaginal deliveries using forceps or vacuum extraction are attributed to inaccurate assessment. This may include an unsuspected cephalopelvic disproportion, incomplete dilatation of the cervix, inadequate anaesthesia, a constriction ring in the uterus, an abnormal position of the head, an unusually large baby or an undiagnosed fetal monsterity. It must be said that the risk of a difficult forceps delivery is inversely proportional to the experience of the operator.

Finally, it has to be emphasized that the second stage of labour must not be regarded by the contemporary obstetrician as the point of no return, and timely recourse to abdominal delivery will save a great deal of dissatisfaction later on.

PUDENDAL NERVE BLOCK: TRANSVAGINAL TECHNIQUE

The pudendal nerve courses from behind the ischial spines, lateral to the pudendal vessels. It supplies the levator ani muscles from its inferior surface, in addition to other deep and superficial perineal muscles. The pudendal nerve also supplies the perineal and vulval skin, with the exception of the anterior two-thirds of the labia majora, which are innervated by the ilioinguinal nerve. Bilateral pudendal nerve block (**Figs 8.1 & 8.2**) is an easy and effective method of pain relief for straightforward forceps delivery, ventouse extraction and the application of forceps for the after-coming head in breech presentation, when epidural anaesthesia has not been used. It is essential to allow 5–7 minutes for the local anaesthetic to block the nerve.

VENTOUSE (VACUUM) EXTRACTION

The forms of assistance required to shorten the second stage of labour constitute a major part of obstetric practice. For many centuries, different tools of a clamp-shaped design have been devised to help the delivery of the fetus, but over the past 300 years, ideas have evolved to utilize the principle of vacuum-assisted traction as a method

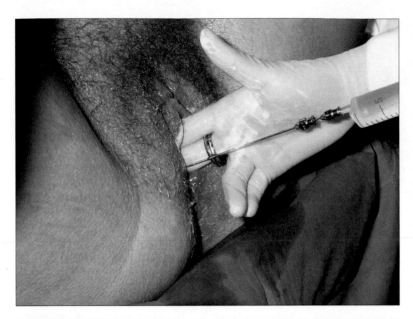

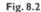

Figs 8.1 & 8.2 Bilateral pudendal nerve block: 10 ml of 0.5–1% lignocaine solution is required to block the pudendal nerve on each side. The solution is injected through a 15-cm 20G needle, which has a guard that is 1 cm shorter than the needle and possesses a small, bulbous end to serve as a guide; the ring attached to the guard is usually worn on the middle finger. The index and middle fingers of the operator's right hand are advanced into the patient's vagina and right vaginal wall, to reach the right ischial spine. In order to gain access to the nerve and deposit the local anaesthetic, the operator aims first at the ischial spine and pierces the attachment of the sacrospinous ligament, just posterior to the tip of the spine, and then directs the needle slightly inferolaterally.

It is essential to avoid intravascular injection; this is accomplished by attempting to aspirate before deposition of the local anaesthetic.

Fig. 8.2

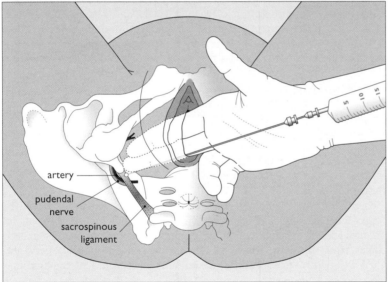

that aids maternal expulsive efforts. The concept seems to have originated from the application of a vacuum to reduce depressed skull fractures in the early 1600s. Whichever design the vacuum cup has received, the most important development has been the successful maintenance of the vacuum.

The proponents of this technique emphasize that no 'space-occupying tools' – that is, forceps blades – are required, and that the principle of delivery relies mainly on skin traction, as opposed to the bony traction of forceps delivery; this mode of assisted delivery results in less trauma to maternal tissues. Its opponents claim that those who promote this concept lack the ability to diagnose the position of the fetal head, and are unable to understand

the mechanics of the obstetric forceps or to apply their blades skilfully, and therefore rely on the pelvic architecture to effect the cardinal movements and the delivery of the baby. Moreover, it is feared that the ability to use the obstetric forceps may vanish. It is, however, self-evident that any technique or expertise should be preserved only if it helps achieve a better outcome.

Clearly, the best result that can be achieved with any method of assisted delivery is dependent on good selection of patients for that procedure and good training. There has been a guarded acceptance of the ventouse extractor in Britain and the United States. However, in Europe and in many parts of the developing world, this instrument has been utilized successfully. Scalp lacerations and cephalohaematoma are the main complications seen with the use of this instrument, but the majority of such mishaps are due to poor selection or insistence on effecting the delivery *per vaginam*, at any cost. It must be remembered, however, that the forceps cause comparable trauma when used in similar situations, and that the appropriate selection of patients is the key to minimizing trauma in operative vaginal delivery of all types.

In addition to providing traction on the head in the occipitoanterior position, vacuum extraction can be successfully used to rotate the head from the occipitoposterior or occipitotransverse position. The instrument can be applied with minimal anaesthesia; even local anaesthesia to the perineum will suffice. In the case of forceps delivery, the minimum required anaesthesia is bilateral pudendal block. Traction, with the ventouse applied to the head as it traverses the perineum, allows a greater control over perineal distension and may even obviate the need for episiotomy (**Figs 8.3–8.17**).

THE OBSTETRIC FORCEPS

The obstetric forceps consist of two blades, designed to produce a grip on the fetal head. Thus the traction, when applied, is exerted mainly on the fetal skull. The instrument

has undergone considerable modification since the original Chamberlen design, and there now exist several different types. The changes in shape of the forceps blade, shank, handle and lock have been dictated by the needs of the individual practitioner when faced with a particular difficulty. In the past, obstetrics was largely concerned with achieving manoeuvrability of the presenting part within any type of pelvis, in an attempt to avoid the then grave consequences of the alternative: caesarean section.

Standard textbooks categorize the types of forceps operation according to the level of the head within the pelvis: high-, mid- and low-cavity forceps delivery. It is an indefensible practice in contemporary obstetrics to perform a high-cavity forceps delivery, and the subject will not be discussed further. A mid-cavity forceps application is said to have been performed when the plane of greatest pelvic dimension accommodates the biparietal diameter of the fetal head, and when the leading bony point is at or just below the ischial spines. When the plane of the biparietal diameter is at or just below the ischial spines, the head is said to be in low cavity. Some obstetricians recommend that even a mid-cavity forceps delivery be performed in the presence of an experienced obstetrician, once the position of the head has been appropriately assessed. In instances of fetal bradycardia, if there is no suspicion of

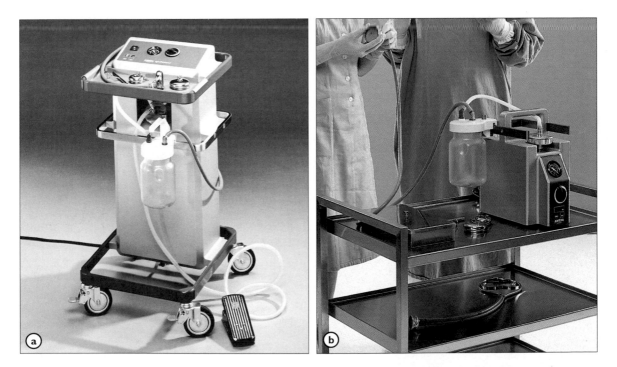

Fig. 8.3a & b Ventouse extraction: the instrument used by the author is Bird's modification of the Malmström Extractor, pictured here. The addition of electrically operated machines for the creation of a vacuum has simplified the procedure. This technique is suitable for the delivery of babies after 35 weeks' gestation. (*Courtesy of Egnell Ameda Ltd., Taunton, UK.*)

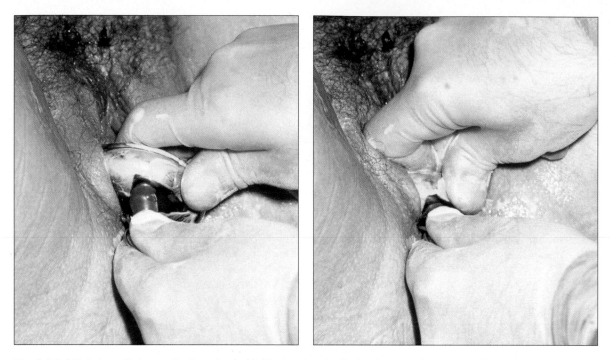

Figs 8.4 & 8.5 As is usually the case in obstetrics, the bladder is catheterized before the operation is started. For the ventouse extraction, the largest cup (7-cm diameter) is always used. The cup is lubricated, introduced into the vagina with the rubber tube attached to it, and applied to the occipital part of the fetal head, preferably with the tube attachment pointing to the occiput as a marker. A digital examination is performed to ensure that the edges of the cup do not impinge on the vaginal skin or cervix, although it must be emphasized that, at least for obstetricians new to this technique, delivery should not be embarked upon if the cervix is not fully dilated.

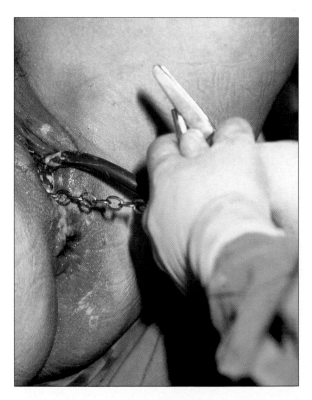

Fig. 8.6 A negative pressure down to $0.2\,kg/cm^2$ is exerted and a repeat digital examination is performed, to ensure that no vaginal or cervical tissue has been sucked into the cup. When this is confirmed, negative pressure down to $0.7–0.8\,kg/cm^2$ is quickly applied, using a mechanical or electrical pump. The operator then waits for 1–2 minutes to allow the chignon (artificial caput) to develop and fill the suction cup.

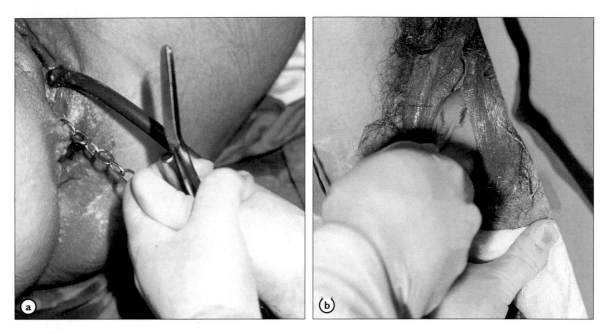

Fig. 8.7a & b During uterine contractions, the patient is encouraged to push and traction is started by pulling on the handle which is attached to the cup by a chain. The operator should be ready to perform an episiotomy if required. The direction of the pull must coincide with the axis of the pelvis throughout, or the vacuum will be interrupted and the cup will slip. **Fig. 8.7b** illustrates the same stage, but with use of the Silastic cup.

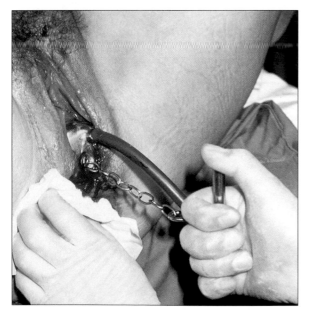

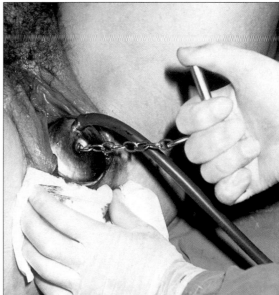

Figs 8.8–8.11 As the descending head distends and stretches the vulva, an episiotomy is performed (**Fig. 8.8**). The direction of traction changes to upwards as the head is brought down to the pelvic outlet. The procedure is performed slowly and steadily, and is usually complete within two or three uterine contractions. Between contractions, traction on the chain is eased slightly, but not so much as to allow the head to slip back. The perineum is supported by being pressed backwards, allowing the face to be delivered without further stretch to the perineal tissues.

Fig. 8.9

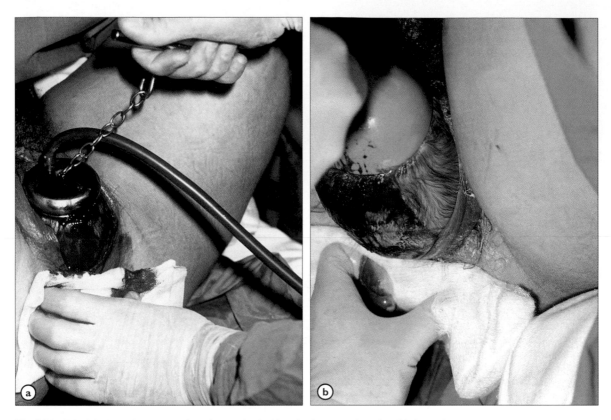

Fig. 8.10a & b (**a**) Upward direction of traction on the fetal head as it crowns the vulva; (**b**) shows the same stage as in (**a**) but a Silastic cup is being used, and in this delivery an episiotomy was not required.

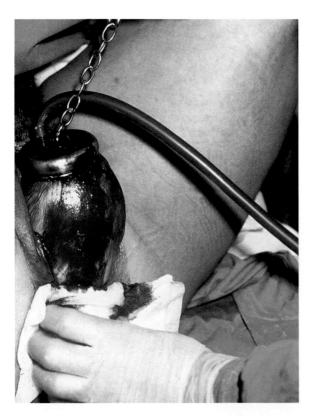

Fig. 8.11 Well-controlled delivery of the head is accomplished. The operator maintains support to the perineum.

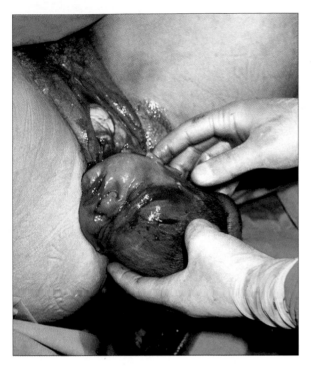

Fig. 8.12 When the head is delivered, restitution to the left occipitoposterior position is completed (in this case, it is 135° clockwise); internal rotation has been successfully accomplished by the baby itself.

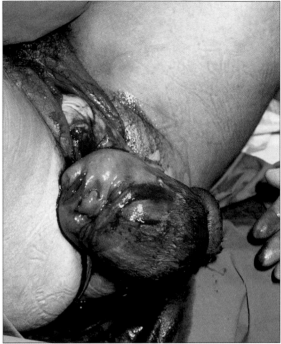

Fig. 8.13 External rotation to the left occipitolateral position follows (in this case, it is 45° anticlockwise), to allow delivery of the shoulders.

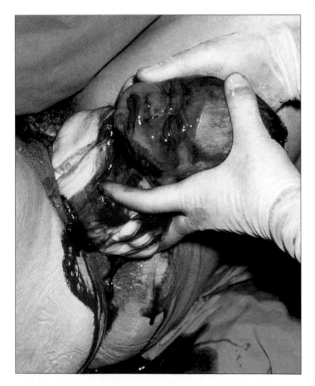

Figs 8.14 & 8.15 The rest of the baby follows.

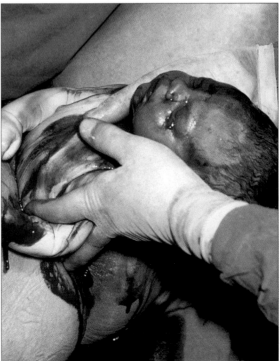

Fig. 8.15

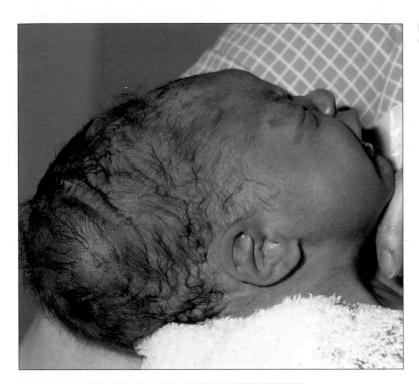

Fig. 8.16 The chignon, seen in profile; it usually disappears with 24–48 hours.

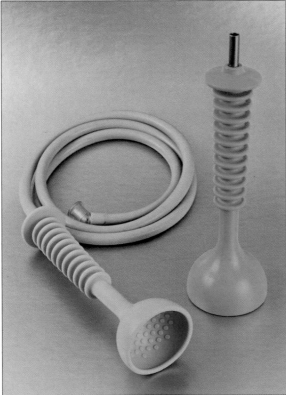

Fig. 8.17 In the new design of vacuum extractor, Silastic cups are used, and the vacuum is generated by an electric motor. This causes less trauma to the head, as no significant chignon is generated by the Silastic cup, which adheres to the head as a result of the negative pressure generated. (*Courtesy of Egnell Ameda Ltd, Taunton, UK.*)

cephalopelvic disproportion, a mid-cavity forceps delivery is an excellent and safe procedure in experienced hands. Nevertheless, it is more traumatic than low-cavity forceps delivery, at least in view of the longer distance the head has to travel down the pelvis, and the consequent longer duration of pressure on the baby's head with the forceps. It is always advisable to refer to the decision-making steps described earlier, to make sure that no factor has been overlooked.

Each half of the obstetric forceps (**Fig. 8.18**) consists of three parts: the blade, the handle and the shank by which these are joined. The shank crosses from one side to the other to join in a recess-like lock. The lock may be English, French or German, depending on the way in which the two halves are assembled: for example, fixed with a screw, or via a simple crossing over of the shanks. The blades possess a curvature from side to side, called the cephalic curve, which cups round the fetal head. The maximum distance between the summits of these curves should not exceed 8 cm, otherwise the blades might slip. The forceps, viewed in profile, have another curve that conforms with the curvature of the lower part of the birth canal; this is referred to as the pelvic curve. The blades of most obstetric forceps are fenestrated, allowing the baby's scalp to protrude through them to give a better grip on the head during traction.

Old textbooks describe 'cephalic application' as opposed to 'pelvic application' of the blades ignoring the position of the fetal head; however, such terminology is outdated and no longer in use.

A pair of forceps should never be applied blindly, even when a dead baby is being delivered, as maternal tissues may be severely damaged.

LOW-CAVITY FORCEPS DELIVERY

Delay in the second stage of labour can occur as a result of maternal fatigue, marginal cephalopelvic disproportion, a rigid perineum or effective epidural anaesthesia, which obtunds the urge to push. Other indications for forceps delivery to shorten the second stage of labour include maternal hypertension, cardiac disease and dural puncture incurred in the course of epidural anaesthesia; in addition, the use of forceps is indicated when profound fetal bradycardia supervenes and progress of the head is rather slow.

The first step in decision making is to ensure that no contraindications to forceps delivery exist.

When the fetal head lies in the occipitoanterior position, any of the following types of forceps may be used: Rhodes (**Fig. 8.19**), Simpson, Neville–Barnes or Haig Ferguson. The last two forceps possess an axis traction handle to help delivery of the head from the mid-cavity; the principle here is that the resultant traction will be exerted along the pelvic axis – the line that passes through the centre of all the pelvic planes. In the usual case of low-cavity forceps delivery, these two forceps are used without their axis traction handles. Apart from the axis traction mechanism, all these four types of forceps are essentially similar: the blades possess a cephalic and a pelvic curve, and are suitable for mid-cavity or low-cavity forceps delivery; they are not suitable for rotation as they traumatize the pelvic tissue if so used, due to the pelvic curve.

Some obstetricians use Wrigley's forceps, which are short-handled, but the tips of the blades impinge sharply on the baby's maxillae and graze the covering skin, especially when moulding is present; these forceps are therefore best avoided.

The position of the head must be carefully assessed. If it lies in the occipitoanterior position, the forceps blades will lock without difficulty. On occasion, if the occipitoposterior position is overlooked, the forceps do not lock easily. When traction is first applied at the beginning of a uterine contraction, the operator must judge the situation: if significant descent is not observed, forceps application is reviewed. When the head lies in the occipitoposterior position, it advances very little, even when strong traction is exerted.

Fig. 8.18 The obstetric forceps (Neville–Barnes).

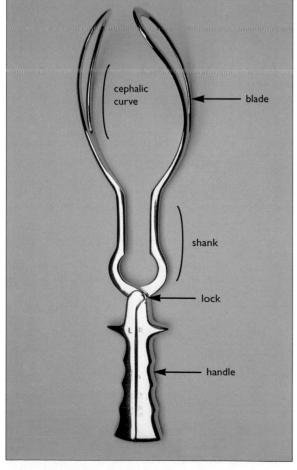

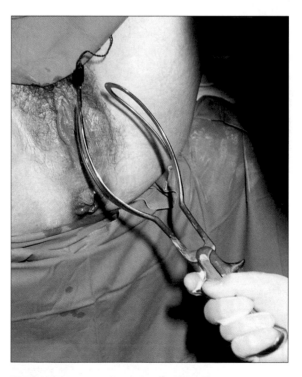

Fig. 8.19 The forceps (Rhodes) are assembled before being used, to ensure both halves are of an identical length.

The patient is anaesthetized with bilateral pudendal nerve block, caudal or epidural anaesthesia, and local sensation is tested; if required, a further dose of local anaesthesia is administered. The bladder is catheterized; a convenient time to do this is while waiting for the bilateral pudendal block to take effect. Occasionally, general anaesthesia may be administered instead.

Figures 8.20–8.36 illustrate the steps in low-cavity forceps delivery.

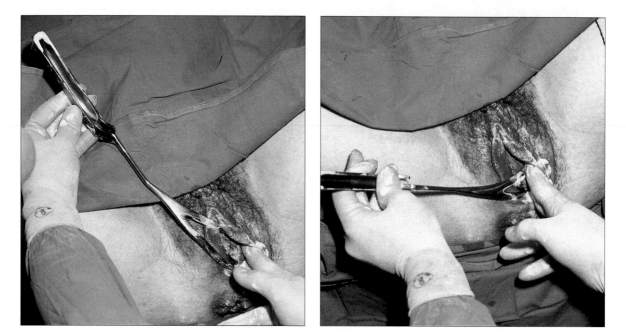

Figs 8.20 & 8.21 Low-cavity forceps delivery: the left handle of the forceps is held in the obstetrician's left hand, in a vertical position (**Fig. 8.20**), and is then swung down to a horizontal level (**Fig. 8.21**), whilst being simultaneously pushed forward into the vagina alongside the fetal head. The forceps blade is guided by the operator's right index and middle fingers, so that it rests on the side of the fetal head.

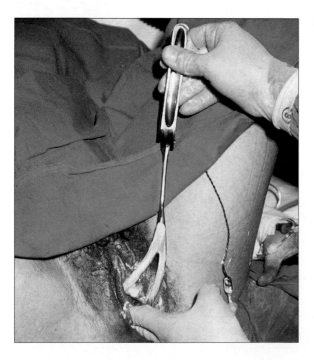

Fig. 8.22 This procedure is repeated similarly on the right side.

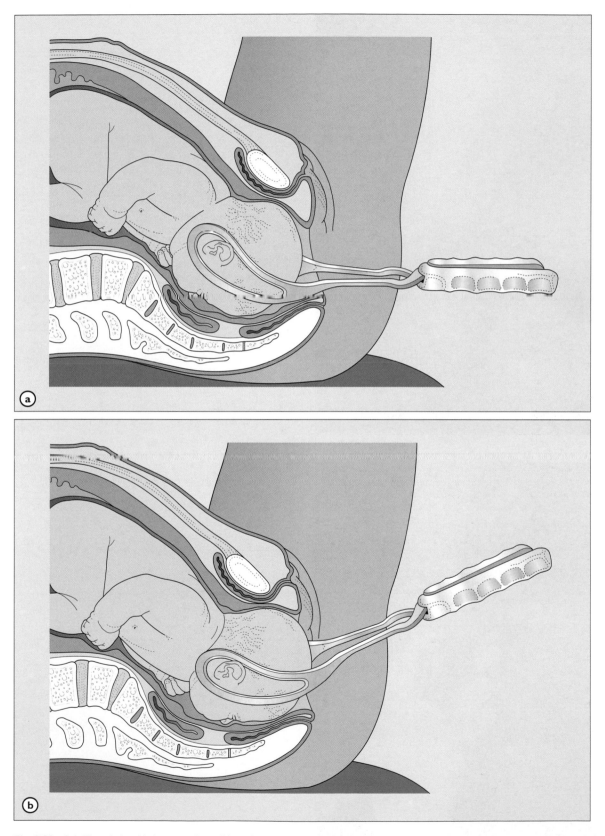

Fig. 8.23a & b The relationship between the pelvic cavity and the pelvic curve of the forceps.

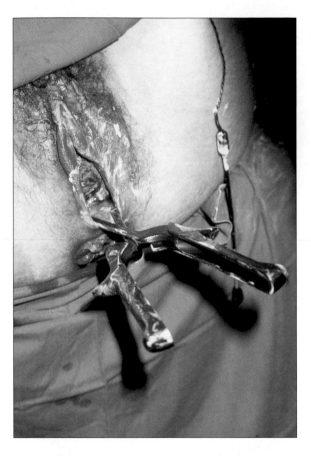

Fig. 8.24 Between contractions, the forceps lock is partially released, to relieve pressure on the fetal head.

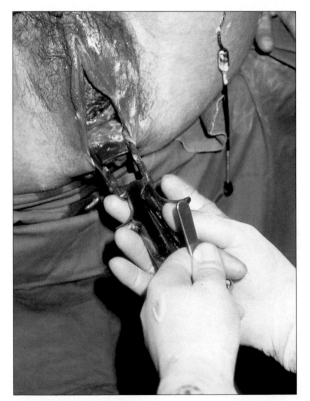

Fig. 8.25 The mother is encouraged to bear down with the onset of the following uterine contraction, and simultaneous traction is applied to the fetal head.

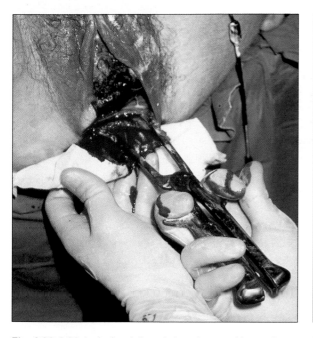

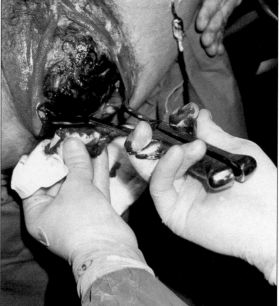

Figs 8.26–8.29 As the head distends the vulva, an episiotomy is performed. During delivery of the head, the perineum is supported with a gauze pad, holding it back and preventing further distension; at the same time, traction is directed upwards away from the perineum.

As soon as the plane of the parietal eminences is delivered, and during the advancement of the head, the forceps are gently dismantled and removed.

Fig. 8.27

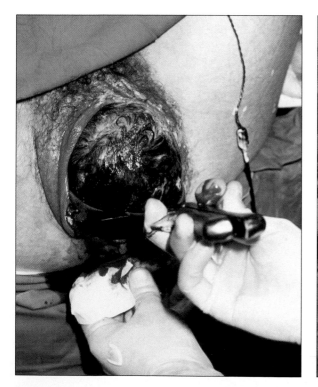

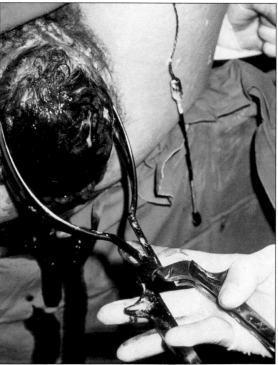

Fig. 8.28

Fig. 8.29

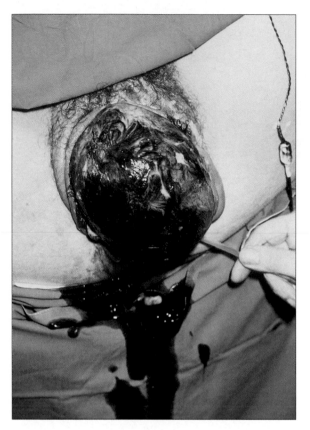

Fig. 8.30 Restitution immediately follows the delivery of the head, undoing the internal rotation, and the occiput is now pointing to 11 o'clock. At this stage, the assistant begins clearing the baby's mouth and nostrils of blood and secretions.

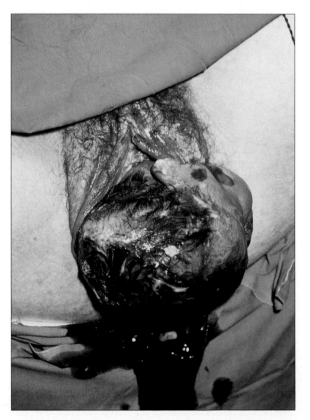

Fig. 8.31 External rotation has taken place with further advancement of the head. This is in response to the rotation of the shoulders, which are now occupying the anteroposterior diameter of the outlet.

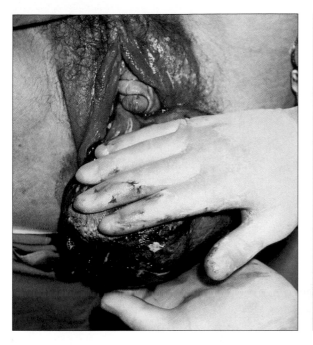

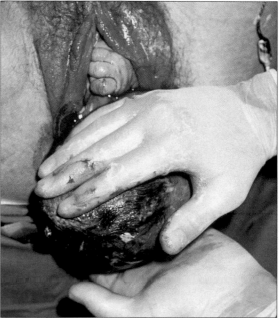

Figs 8.32 & 8.33 With the onset of the following contraction, the head is held between the operator's hands and traction, with pressure directed posteriorly (downwards), is applied to help the delivery of the anterior shoulder. The baby's right hand is visible, as here the right arm lies across the baby's thorax and is lower in the pelvis than the left shoulder.

Fig. 8.33

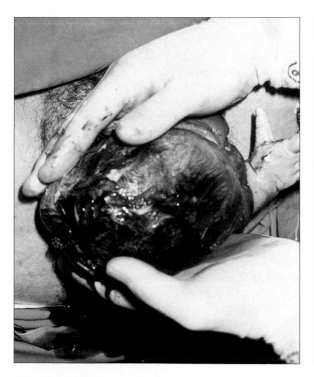

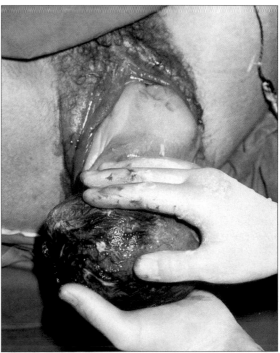

Fig. 8.34 The right arm and the posterior shoulder are therefore eased out and delivered first, by raising the baby's head using slight traction.

Fig. 8.35 Further traction on the baby is then applied; the operator holds the head between both hands and pulls in a downwards direction to deliver the anterior shoulder.

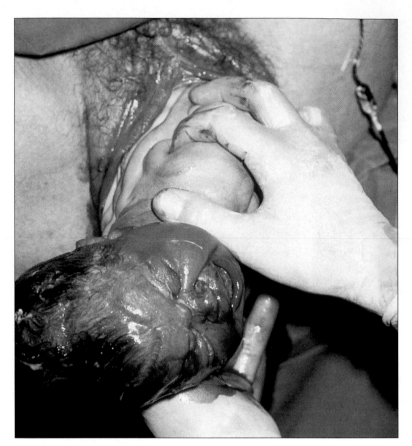

Fig. 8.36 The rest of the baby is easily delivered.

KJELLAND'S FORCEPS DELIVERY

Christian Kjelland (1871–1941) designed the forceps (**Fig. 8.37a**) that bear his name during the first 10 years of his medical career; he published his paper describing the forceps in 1916. The introduction of these forceps gave rise to a variety of controversial claims, and their role was, and still is, doubted by many. They were designed to facilitate the delivery of the high head – that is, delivery of a baby whose head lies at the level of the pelvic inlet.

Kjelland recognized that straight forceps, like those designed by Chamberlen and Smellie, allow rotation of the presenting part within the vagina, While forceps such as those of Neville–Barnes, Simpson and many others are not suitable for rotation in view of their pronounced pelvic curve. Kjelland's forceps have been described as straight, but the blades are in fact at a lower level than the shank when seen in profile (**Fig. 8.37b**) and therefore possess a slight pelvic curve, which helps the delivery of the head along the pelvic axis.

The instrument is composed of two blades with handles, which are linked by the shank. When the forceps are assembled, the blades converge at their shanks, the surfaces of which are flat and can be fitted together, held by a sliding lock that points anteriorly; this allows greater mobility of the blades without compromising the stability of the forceps. As in most types of forceps, the blades are fenestrated and rounded, so that when the soft tissue of the head bulges through, they offer further grip. The handles have two sets of shoulders, the proximal and the distal, respectively those nearest the operator and those farthest away. On each of the distal shoulders, there is a knob that points to the same side as the sliding lock. This helps the obstetrician to determine the direction of application of each blade, as these knobs, and therefore the lock, must be directed towards the occiput (**Fig. 8.38**). The proximal shoulders help to exert rotational force on the fetal head, whilst the distal shoulders serve as points against which traction is applied.

DEEP TRANSVERSE POSITION OF THE HEAD
Direct Application of the Blades
The second stage of the labour shown in **Figures 8.39–8.58** was arrested with the head in the right occipitolateral position.

Application of the Blades by the Wandering Method
In the delivery shown in **Figures 8.59–8.67**, the head has not advanced beyond the level of the ischial spines, and its internal rotation has been arrested in the left occipitotransverse position.

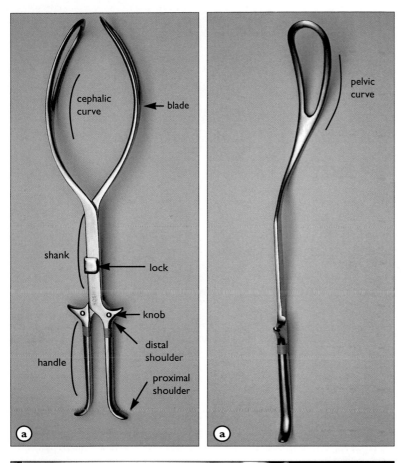

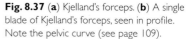

Fig. 8.37 (**a**) Kjelland's forceps. (**b**) A single blade of Kjelland's forceps, seen in profile. Note the pelvic curve (see page 109).

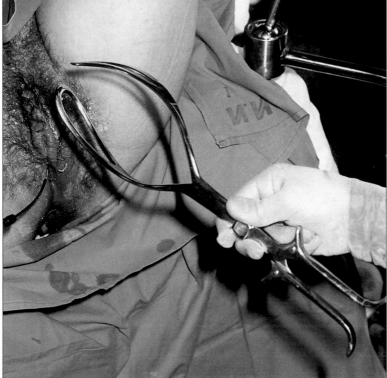

Fig. 8.38 The Kjelland's forceps are assembled to check that both halves are of exactly the same length, and correctly locked. This step also helps the beginner to ascertain which blade will be the anterior one, because, before application, the knobs on the shanks are directed towards the occiput.

The position of the patient should be checked to ensure that her buttocks are clear of the edge of the table, to allow manoeuverability of the forceps blades.

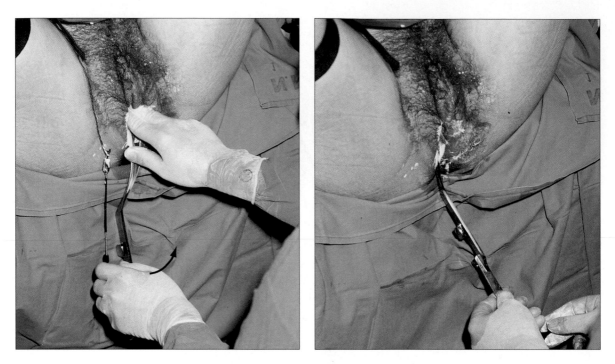

Figs 8.39 & 8.40 The anterior blade is introduced first. The handle is held vertically in the operator's left hand, with the knob on the distal shoulder and, therefore, the lock pointing towards the occiput. The blade is then guided by the right index and middle fingers to slip gently over the baby's head, through an upward swing (arrow).

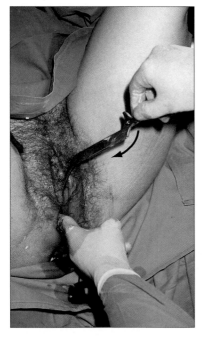

Fig. 8.41 The posterior blade is likewise inserted, but here the handle, which is held vertically, is swung from above in a downwards and inwards direction (arrow).

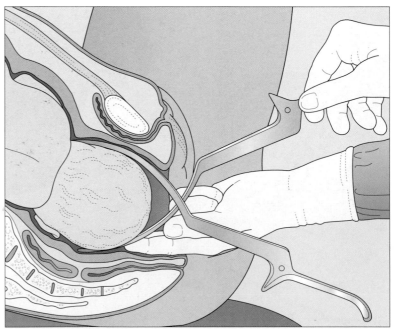

Fig. 8.42 Sagittal section through the pelvis, showing the relationship between the Kjelland's forceps blades, the baby's head and the pelvic landmarks.

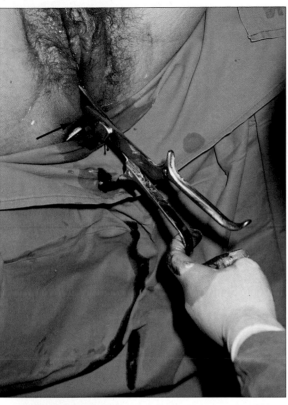

Fig. 8.43 When the forceps are locked, they are seen to press markedly on the perineum (arrow), and clearly indicate posterior asynclitism (posterior parietal bone presentation), as the handle of the posterior blade looks longer than that of the anterior blade.

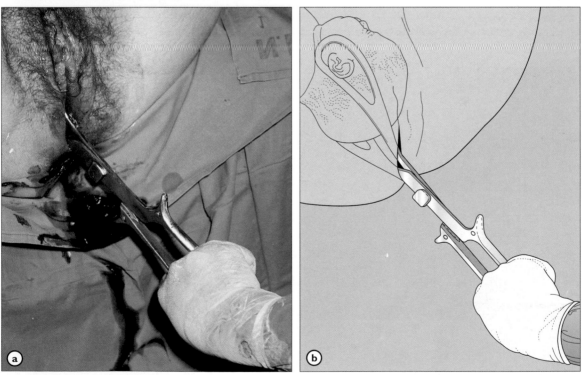

Fig. 8.44a & b The forceps are held by the proximal shoulders to effect rotation between contractions. (Note the way the proximal shoulders of the forceps are held in **Fig. 8.56**.)

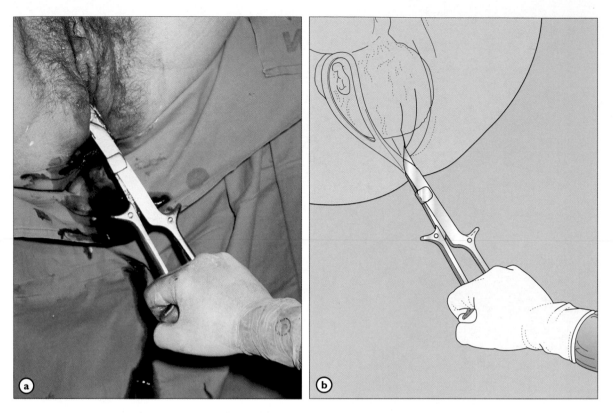

Fig. 8.45a & b Clockwise rotation from the right occipitolateral to the occipitoanterior position is accomplished. Note that, at this stage, no attempt has been made to correct asynclitism by trying to adjust the length of the forceps handles. When the rotation is successfully completed, asynclitism will be corrected at the same time.

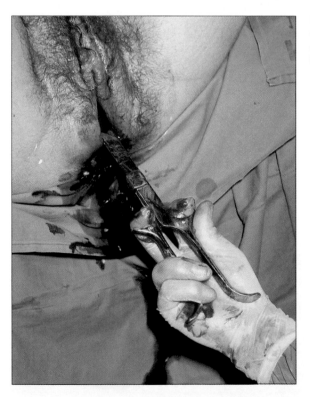

Fig. 8.46 The handles are held by the distal shoulders, the operator begins traction, at which stage asynclitism has been corrected with the rotation, and the blade's shoulders are seen to be level.

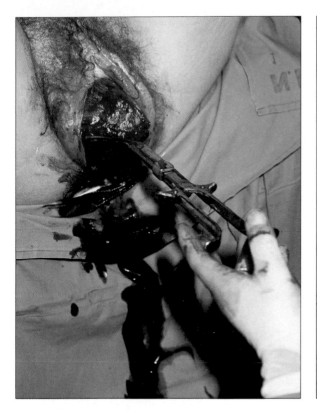

Fig. 8.47 As the head stretches the vulva, an episiotomy is performed

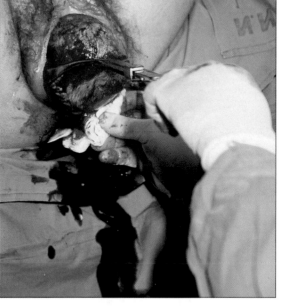

Fig. 8.48 Traction is initially downwards and then upwards, to effect extension of the head.

Fig. 8.49 When the face starts to appear, the forceps are gently dismantled.

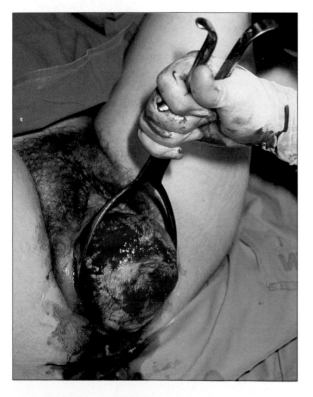

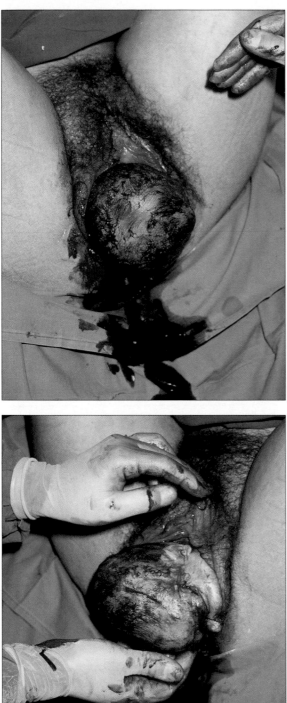

Figs 8.50–8.52 Restitution immediately follows, from the occipitoanterior position all the way back to the right occipitoposterior position (135°).

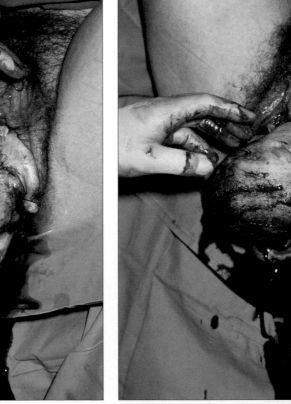

Fig 8.51

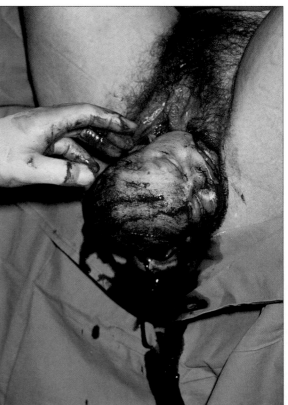

Fig. 8.52

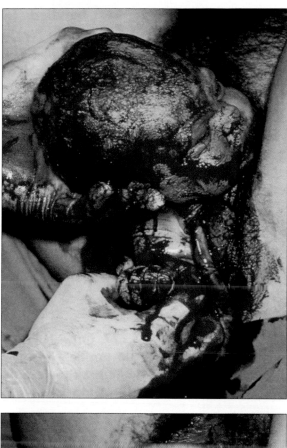

Fig. 8.53 External rotation from the right occipitoposterior position to the right occipitotransverse position (45°) has occurred, because of the alignment of the bisacromial diameter with the anteroposterior diameter of the outlet. In this case, the posterior shoulder is delivered first.

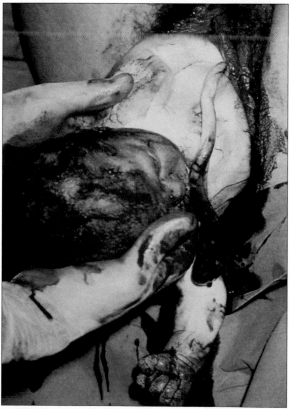

Fig. 8.54 The anterior shoulder and the rest of the body follows.

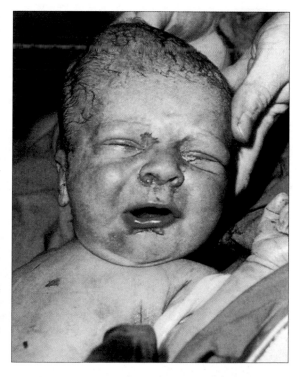

Fig. 8.55 The effect of posterior asynclitism on the shape of the newborn's head. Asynclitism is the lateral flexion of the fetal head, which represents its adaptation to the shape of the pelvis. It is a common finding in a mild form, but occasionally it may be severe, with marked overlap of the parietal bones.

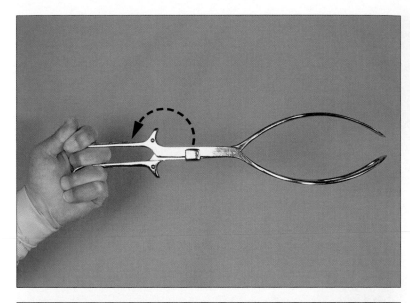

Fig. 8.56 The way in which Kjelland's forceps are handled to effect rotation (arrow) is very important: the operator must not grip the handles in such a way that they are brought close together. The index and ring fingers are hooked over the proximal shoulders, with the middle finger placed between the handles to prevent them coming too close together, and thus ensuring that the head is not compressed excessively by the blades.

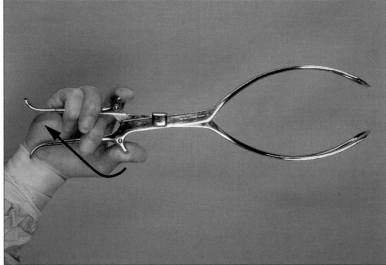

Figs 8.57 & 8.58 Other techniques used to effect rotation include the application of digital pressure against the distal shoulders to effect clockwise (arrow) (**Fig. 8.57**) or anticlockwise (arrow) (**Fig. 8.58**) rotation of the head.

Fig. 8.58

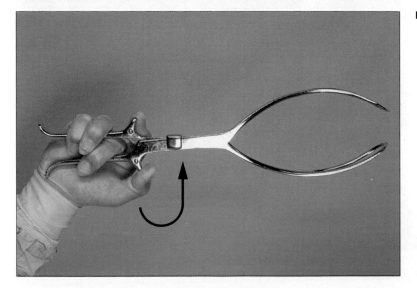

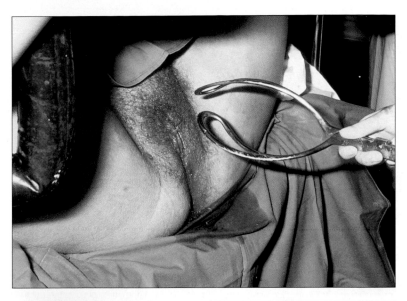

Fig. 8.59 The forceps are assembled to check that the two halves are of exactly the same length, and they are held in the position in which they are to fit the fetal head, with their knobs facing the left side of the patient.

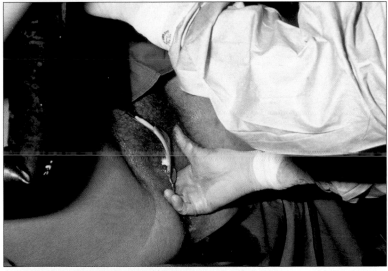

Fig. 8.60 The anterior blade is introduced first: the handle is held vertically in the operator's left hand, with the knob on the distal shoulder pointing towards the floor. The blade is guided by the right index and middle fingers to slip over the baby's occiput, and then round the head, to rest on the baby's anterior temple. The knob now points towards the left side of the pelvis, where the occiput lies.

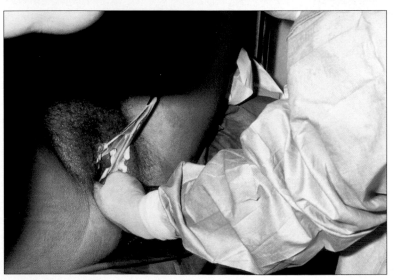

Fig. 8.61 The posterior blade is inserted by direct application.

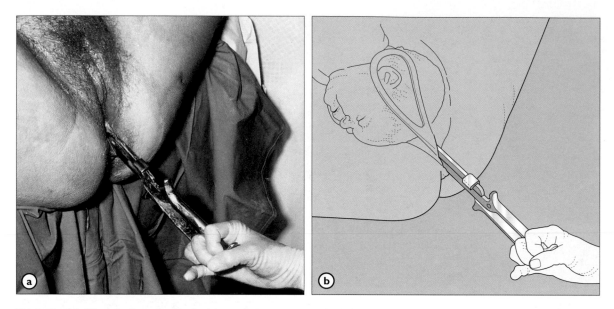

Fig. 8.62a & b When the forceps are locked, they are seen to press markedly over the perineum, which clearly shows posterior asynclitism, as the handle of the posterior blade looks longer than that of the anterior blade. The forceps are held by the proximal shoulders to effect rotation between contractions.

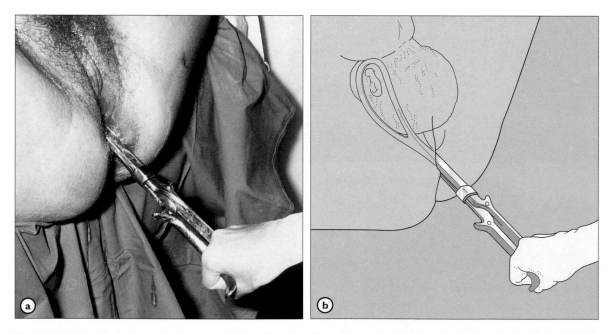

Fig. 8.63a & b Anticlockwise rotation from the left occipitolateral to the occipitoanterior position is accomplished, and no attempt has been made to correct asynclitism at this stage.

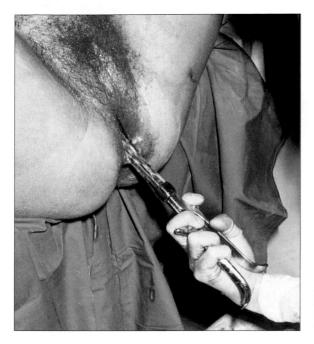

Fig. 8.64 The operator starts traction, holding the handles by the distal shoulders, at which stage asynclitism has been corrected with the rotation.

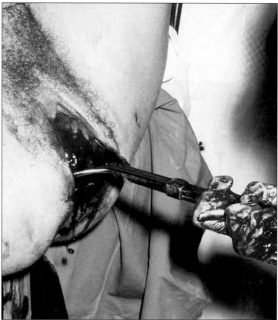

Fig. 8.65 As the head stretches the vulva, an episiotomy is performed.

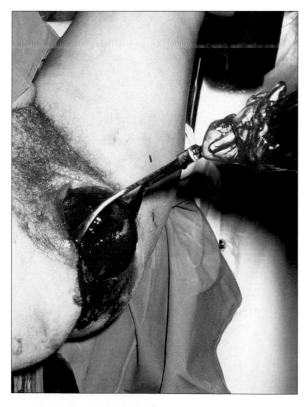

Fig. 8.66 Traction is initially downwards, and then upwards to effect extension of the head.

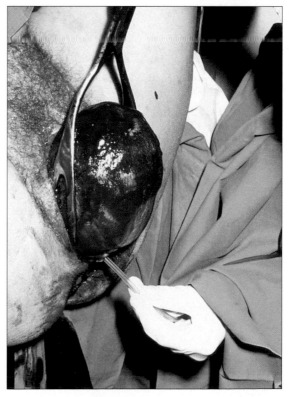

Fig. 8.67 When the face begins to appear, the forceps are gently dismantled, and the assistant starts mouth and nasal suction to clear these orifices of blood and secretions.

DELIVERY OF THE OCCIPITOPOSTERIOR POSITION

The forceps are assembled with the lock and the knobs facing posteriorly (towards the floor), in the position in which they will lock when applied to the fetal head. **Figures 8.68–8.79** illustrate this method of delivery.

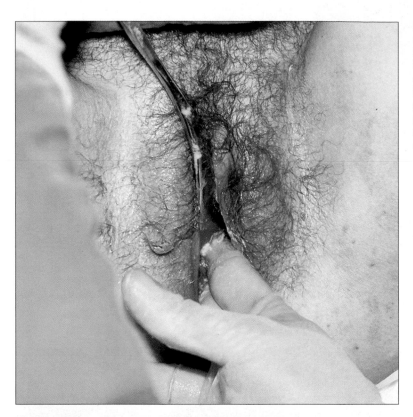

Figs 8.68 & 8.69 Delivery of the occipitoposterior position: the left. and then the right blade is applied, as in the introduction of Simpson's or any other ordinary forceps, but with the pelvic curve facing downwards. The forceps blade is gently guided by the appropriate hand into position at the side of the baby's head, by arching the handle from above in a downward movement, with an inward push.

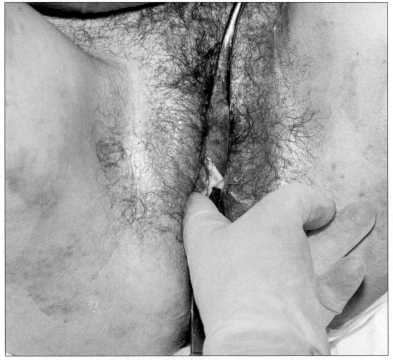

Fig. 8.69

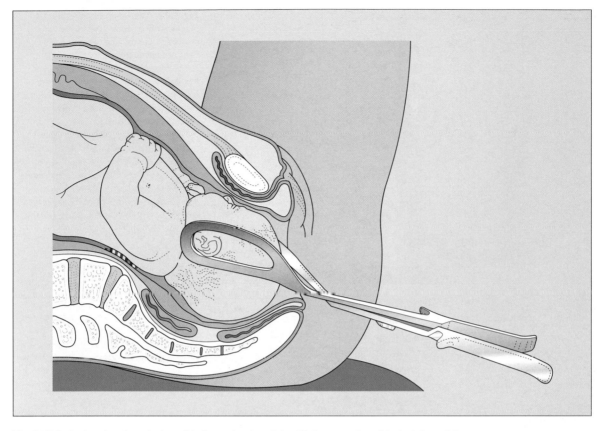

Fig. 8.70 Sagittal section through the pelvis, illustrating the relationship between the pelvis, the baby and the applied Kjelland's forceps, pictured below in **Fig. 8.71**

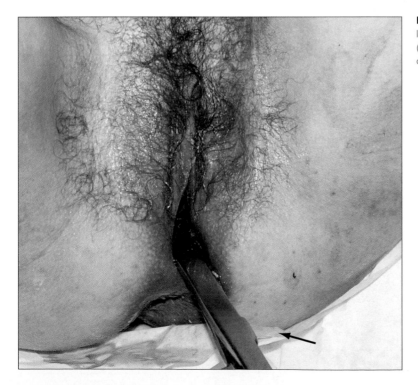

Fig. 8.71 Kjelland's forceps in position, locked on the baby's head. Note the lock (arrow) is pointing downwards, towards the occiput.

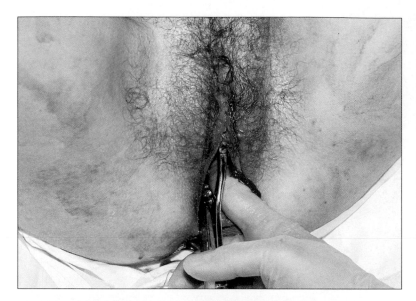

Fig. 8.72 When the uterus relaxes between contractions, the forceps are rotated clockwise. The head now lies in the right occipitolateral position. It should be remembered that Kjelland's forceps are held by the proximal shoulders during rotation, and that rotation would have been anticlockwise, had the head been in the left occipitoposterior position.

Halfway through the rotation, the position of the head is checked to ensure that the sagittal suture has been successfully moved to occupy the transverse diameter of the pelvic cavity; note that the operator is checking with his right index finger for the position of the sagittal suture and the anterior fontanelle.

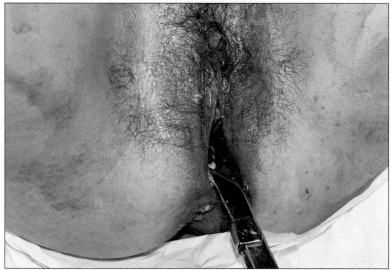

Figs 8.73 & 8.74 Rotation of the head to the occipitoanterior position is completed, and the sagittal suture now occupies the anteroposterior diameter of the pelvic cavity once again. Traction on the fetal head is exerted as the operator pulls on the distal shoulders of the Kjelland's forceps.

Fig. 8.74

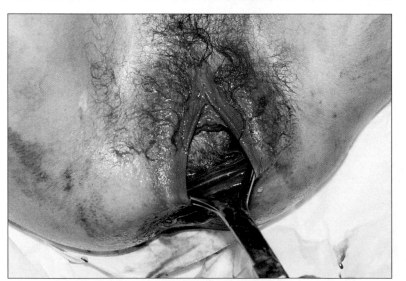

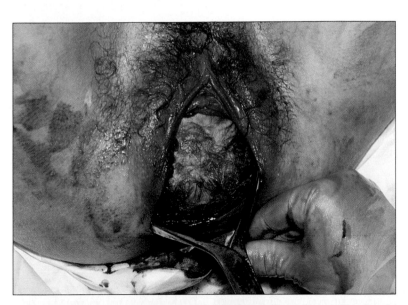

Fig. 8.75 When the head distends the vulva, an episiotomy is performed.

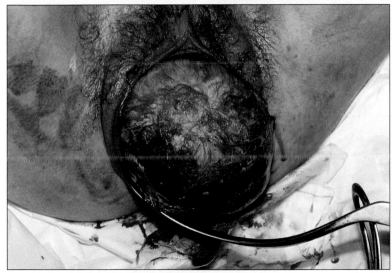

Fig. 8.76 As the head is delivered, the forceps are dismantled and restitution immediately follows, with the occiput rotating back to the right occipitoposterior position (135°) (not shown).

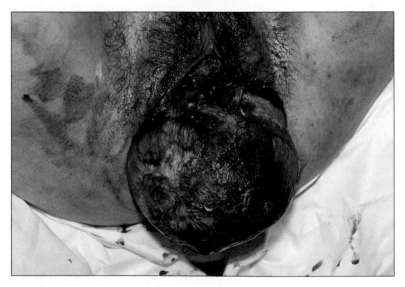

Fig. 8.77 External rotation to the right occipitolateral position (45°) follows with the next contraction, as the bisacromial diameter becomes aligned with the anteroposterior diameter of the outlet.

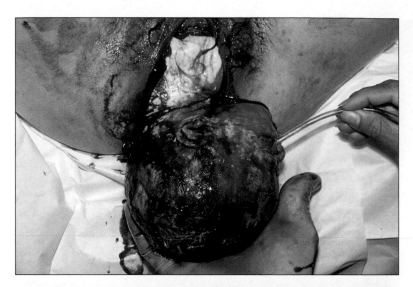

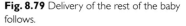

Fig. 8.78 Suction clearance of the mouth and nostrils is performed at this stage.

Fig. 8.79 Delivery of the rest of the baby follows.

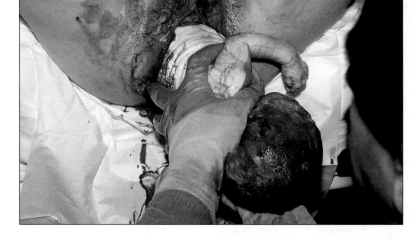

MANUAL ROTATION OF THE HEAD AND FORCEPS DELIVERY

The claims of extensive injuries resulting from Kjelland's forceps rotation and delivery are controversial, and these injuries can be largely avoided by a rigorous selection of patients and adequate training. However, some obstetricians do hold extreme views on the subject that have led them to dispense completely with the Kjelland's forceps in their units and to adopt, instead, the technique of manual rotation of the head and forceps delivery. Claims for a lower incidence of fetal injury may be accepted, despite the fact that there exists no detailed controlled and randomized study to confirm the superiority of such a technique over rotational forceps or ventouse delivery in well-selected cases.

The position of the head must be assessed carefully, as in any other operative vaginal delivery. The key to successful diagnosis of the position of the fetal head starts with abdominal examination, which is sometimes overlooked. Abdominal palpation helps to determine the fetal lie and presentation, the position of the back, and the proportion of the fetal head still palpable *per abdomen*, above the pelvic brim; this pays dividends when the findings at vaginal examination require further interpretation. During vaginal examination, in particular when the obstetrician's help is sought, the landmarks of the presenting part are totally obscured by advanced caput succedaneum and a degree of asynclitism, which may even obscure the sagittal suture. In these patients, it is useful to pass two fingers to the side of the fetal head, attempting to feel for the ear; this can help to ascertain the location of the sagittal suture, and sometimes even the position of the occiput.

Technique

The technique of manual rotation of the head requires the operator to introduce his or her hand into the vagina, and to hold the baby's head to effect its rotation. This is performed after the urinary bladder has been catheterized, and when the bilateral pudendal block, or other type of anaesthesia, has taken effect. As supination of the forearm is a more efficient and stronger movement than pronation, the operator's hand is cupped around the fetal head, with the thumb and the index finger arched round the occiput. The operator's right hand is used to correct the right occipitoposterior and right occipitolateral positions of the head (**Fig. 8.80a & b**), and the left hand is used to correct the left occipitoposterior and left occipitolateral positions of the head, so that supination is the movement used to effect rotation; this is performed between contractions. Sometimes it is necessary to dislodge the head slightly upwards (cephalad) before turning it.

As the head rotates, the operator helps the movement by using the other hand on the lower abdomen to apply concomitant pressure on the anterior shoulder, thus promoting whole-body rotation. When this movement is complete, a mid-cavity forceps delivery is performed, using a pair of Simpson's, Rhodes', Haig Ferguson's or Neville–Barnes' forceps. The procedure is exactly the same as that used in low-cavity forceps delivery, with one exception: initial traction is directed more caudally until the head reaches the pelvic floor, at which point the direction of traction is curved upwards (or anteriorly).

Occasionally, rotation of the head to the occipitoanterior position is difficult to achieve and, because of the shape of the pelvis at least, the operator can rotate the head only to the occipitoposterior position. In these circumstances, the application of the forceps and the subsequent delivery of the head with face-to-pubis is a possible course of action. However, because of the maternal soft-

tissue injury that accompanies face-to-pubis delivery, it cannot be justified, except where:
- Fetal distress is present.
- The attendant is not skilled in Kjelland's forceps rotation delivery.
- There is no indication of cephalopelvic disproportion. It has to be remembered that more forceful traction with the forceps is required to deliver the head when it lies in the occipitoposterior position and is associated with slow advancement of the head. Such force results in marked facial bruising and laceration. The extent of maternal soft-tissue damage seen in these deliveries, especially the extension of the episiotomy up to the vaginal fornix, may necessitate even general anaesthesia to facilitate the repair.

Another modification of this technique, sometimes used by the author, is as follows. The right hand is always used to rotate the head. When manual rotation of the head to the occipitoanterior position is completed, the hand is kept in the vagina to guide the forceps blade (the left blade), which, once introduced, will usually arrest the tendency of the head to slip back. If the position of the occiput is right posterior, the hand is introduced in pronation so that the index and thumb arch over the occiput and, when the clockwise rotation is completed, the hand will lie on the left side of the head.

In the case of the left occipitoposterior position, the right hand is introduced to take an exaggerated supination position, with the operator's thumb and index finger forming an arch over the occiput, and the fingers over the left side of the head. When the anticlockwise rotation is completed, the fingers of the right hand will be against the left side of the head, and therefore can then be used to guide the left forceps blade into position.

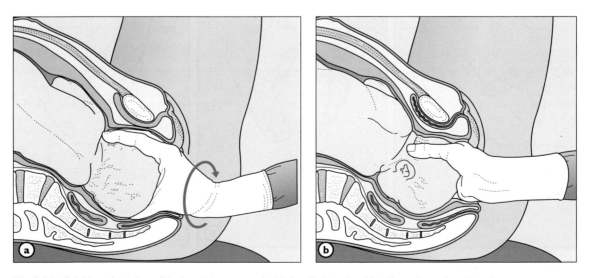

Fig. 8.80a & b Manual rotation of the head: the operator's right hand is introduced into the vagina and positioned in pronation, so that the index finger and thumb arch over the occiput, and the other fingers lie on the parietal bone to assist in grasping the head. The head is then successfully rotated to the occipitoanterior position. The arrow indicates the clockwise direction of the manoeuvre.

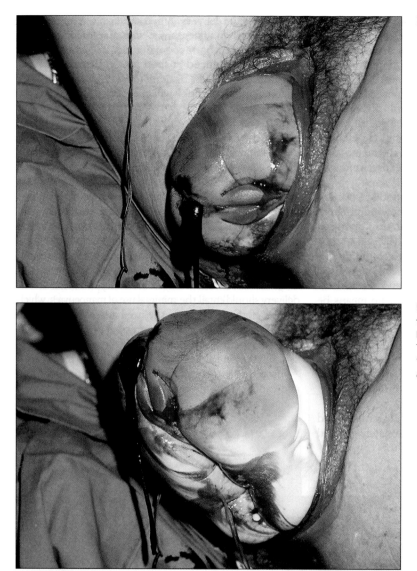

Fig. 9.4

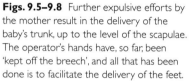

Figs. 9.5–9.8 Further expulsive efforts by the mother result in the delivery of the baby's trunk, up to the level of the scapulae. The operator's hands have, so far, been 'kept off the breech', and all that has been done is to facilitate the delivery of the feet.

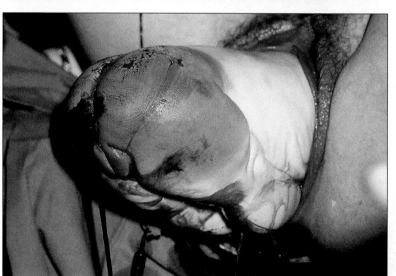

Fig. 9.6

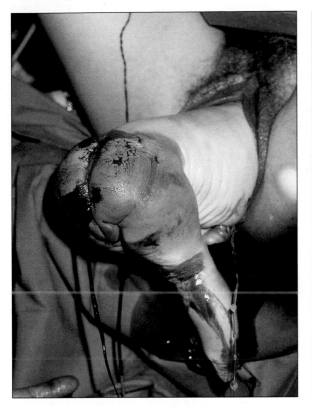

Fig. 9.7

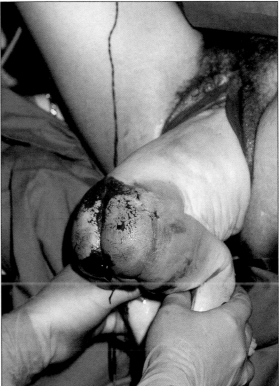

Fig. 9.8

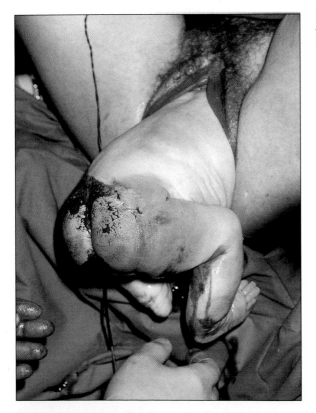

Fig. 9.9 The obstetrician makes sure the baby's back is upward all the time. The tip of the right scapula has just appeared, which indicates that the shoulders have descended further into the pelvis.

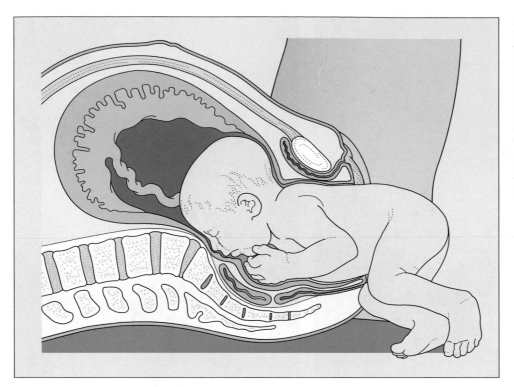

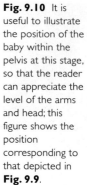

Fig. 9.10 It is useful to illustrate the position of the baby within the pelvis at this stage, so that the reader can appreciate the level of the arms and head; this figure shows the position corresponding to that depicted in **Fig. 9.9**.

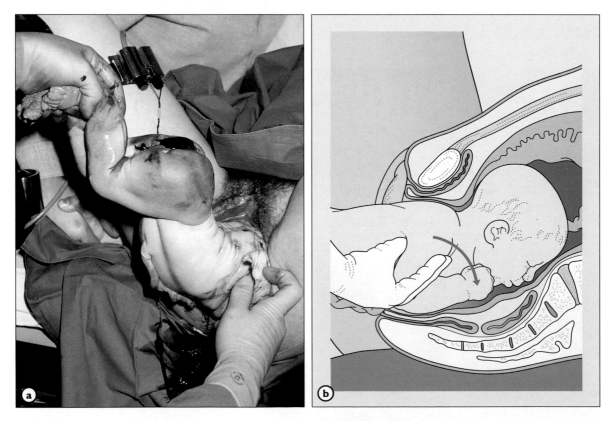

Fig. 9.11a & b As the anterior shoulder descends into the pelvis, the operator holds both ankles with the left hand and inserts the right index and middle fingers into the vagina. He then delivers the right arm by pressing it from above downwards, towards the cubital fossa, sweeping it across the baby's chest to be extracted from under the pubic rami.

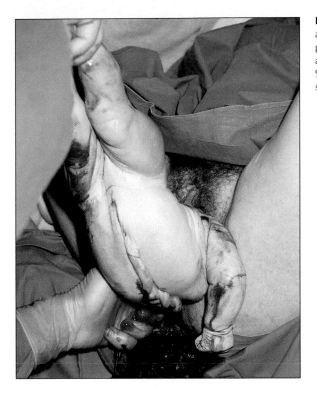

Fig. 9.12 The process is then repeated on the other side, where access to the left arm is gained from the posterior part of the pelvic outlet, because the hollow of the sacrum allows easier access. Alternatively, the obstetrician may rotate the baby's trunk 90° clockwise, to gain access to the left arm from under the pubic symphysis.

is at the pelvic floor and the fetal heart rate shows profound bradycardia; here the performance of an episiotomy and breech extraction are thoroughly justified, particularly when the operator is satisfied that no obvious fetopelvic disproportion exists. If one or both feet are already in the vagina, it or they are grasped by the ankle and traction is applied to bring the buttock further down the pelvis.

PINARD'S MANOEUVRE
In the case of frank breech, with the breech impacted by extended legs, Pinard's manoeuvre is applied (**Fig. 9.13**). Sometimes the legs are well splinted in a frank breech presentation and may halt the progress of labour. They can be delivered by the operator, who supports the fetal thigh with his index and middle fingers, pressing at the popliteal fossa and simultaneously effecting a gentle but firm abduction at the hip joint. This composite manoeuvre will result in flexion at the knee and the easy delivery of the foot, which is pulled out of the vagina. Sometimes it is necessary first to disimpact the breech, which may require general or adequate conduction anaesthesia.

LÖVSET'S MANOEUVRE
The term 'nuchal arm' describes a fetal position that includes an extended shoulder, a flexed elbow and a forearm located behind the head. It is an infrequent complication of breech births, and may be overcome with the help of Lövset's manoeuvre. The aim of the manoeuvre

when used in this situation is to steady the fetal arm against the contracted and retracted uterine wall, allowing the operator's finger to assist flexion and delivery (**Figs 9.14–9.22**).

CEPHALIC COMPLICATIONS
Difficulties may arise when the fetal head is extended or too big to engage. Time is at a premium, and response to a call for help may come too late. Any obstetrician who embarks on the delivery of a breech has therefore to be prepared for this event. The operator's right hand is introduced into the vagina, to make an assessment of the situation and to identify the reason for this difficulty. An incompletely dilated cervix is probably the most common cause in preterm breeches, whereas in term breeches an extended head or hydrocephalus may be responsible. In the absence of a grossly enlarged head or incomplete cervical dilatation, an attempt is made with the left hand (*per abdomen*) to rotate and negotiate the head through the pelvic brim.

It has to be borne in mind that anoxic brain damage may occur within 3–5 minutes if delivery is not effected. Valuable time should not be wasted in trying to apply forceps on such a high head, as this will inevitably fail. Instead, a posterior vaginal wall retractor should be introduced, in an attempt to expose the baby's nostrils and clear the air passages, allowing the baby to breathe. This is the time to reassess the situation and to plan further action. If the cervix is incompletely dilated, a posterior wall retractor is placed *in situ* and the cervix is incised in the midline, posteriorly, and delivery is effected. In the absence of hydrocephalus, another attempt is made bimanually to increase flexion of the head, and to negotiate it through the oblique or transverse diameter of the inlet, completing the delivery by applying forceps to the after-coming head, when it has descended sufficiently into the pelvis.

Should these efforts fail, a form of decompression of the head would be necessary, as the baby would have died by this time. In the case of hydrocephalus, decompression via a perforation aimed at the foramen magnum may be required.

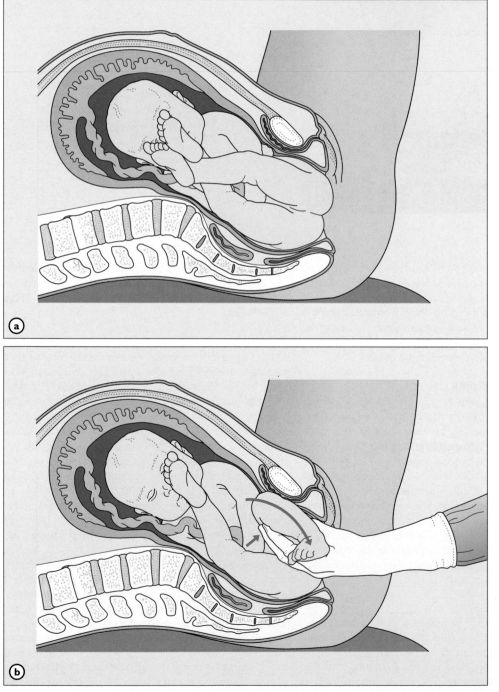

Fig. 9.13a & b
Pinard's manoeuvre: this involves the abduction of the thigh at the hip joint, which results in flexion of the knee and brings the foot within reach for traction and delivery.

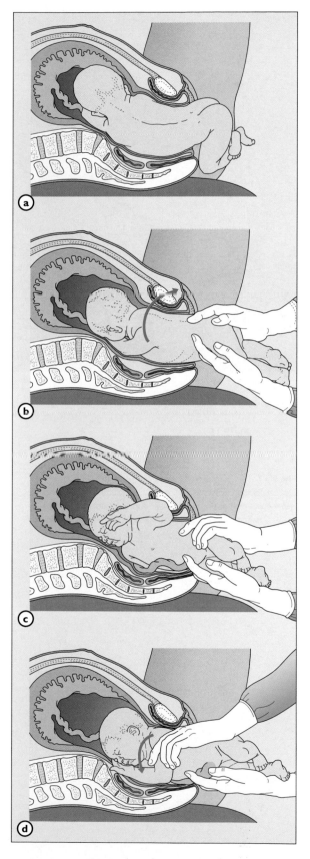

Fig. 9.14a–d Lövset's manoeuvre: this involves rotating the body of the baby so that the posterior shoulder rotates to the front, in a spiral, downward path. The posterior shoulder, which becomes anterior, is then delivered from under the symphysis pubis. This manoeuvre is particularly useful for the delivery of the extended arm or of the nuchal arm. The rotation of the baby with its back kept upwards facilitates the adduction of the extended arm, which slips medially.

Lövset's manoeuvre, in the delivery of a right sacrolateral position, in which the anterior shoulder is the right shoulder (**Fig. 9.14a**), involves holding the baby by the buttocks, exerting slight steady traction, and firstly rotating the baby 180° clockwise (abdomen towards the maternal right thigh) (**Fig. 9.14b & c**), to allow the posterior shoulder to appear under the pubic symphysis and the right shoulder to occupy the hollow of the sacrum. The operator's left index and middle fingers are slipped along the baby's arm, applying a firm but gentle pressure on the cubital fossa and not against the arm, thus encouraging a movement of flexion and adduction (**Fig. 9.14d**).

Owing to the shape of the pelvic cavity, the posterior shoulder usually descends to a lower level than the anterior shoulder. Therefore, after the first rotation of 180°, it will be easier to gain access to the 'new' posterior shoulder, because of the hollow of the sacrum. If the posterior shoulder is not delivered, trunk rotation is performed 180° in the opposite direction, together with traction, to bring the posterior shoulder to lie anteriorly, under the symphysis pubis.

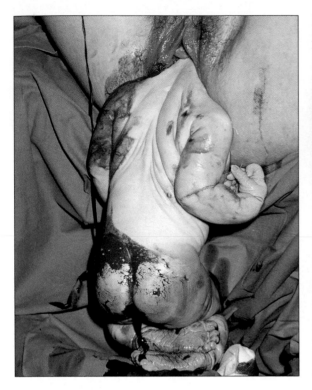

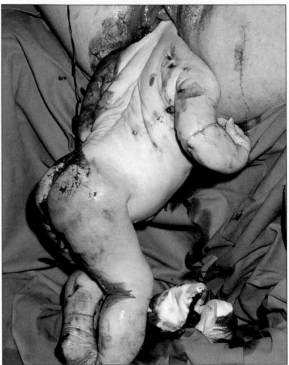

Fig. 9.15 After delivery of the arms, the baby is allowed to hang for about 1 minute, in order to exert traction on the head through body weight, until the nuchal hair line becomes visible. This indicates that the head has descended sufficiently down the pelvis.

Fig. 9.16 Further descent of the after-coming head and its negotiation of the pelvic cavity. The nuchal hair line becomes visible and the baby has actually moved from its previous position in **Fig. 9.15**.

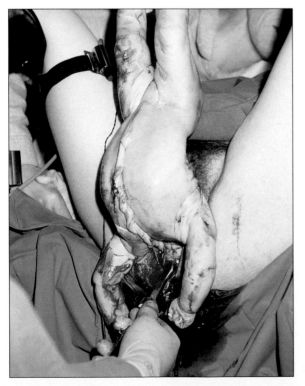

Fig. 9.17 The baby is lifted upwards by the ankles from the vertical position, towards the mother's abdomen in a 135° curve, and the assistant supports the ankles in this position.

At this juncture, if the operator feels that the umbilical cord is tight, he can divide it between clamps.

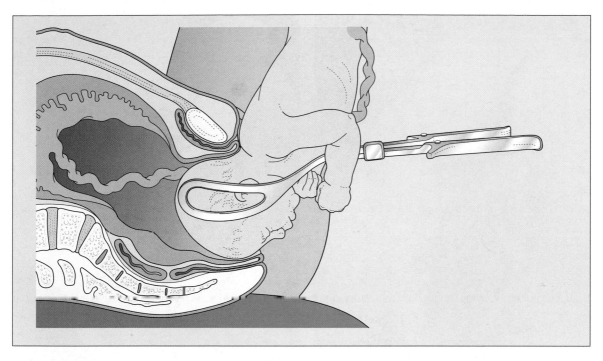

Figs 9.18–9.21 Forceps such as Kjelland's are applied to the after-coming head (in the United States, Piper's forceps are more commonly used), and steady and well-controlled delivery of the fetal head is achieved by initially pulling downwards and then slowly and gently directing the traction upwards. As the mouth and nostrils become visible at the perineum, they are cleared by suction. The baby's head is allowed to rest on the perineum and a gentle traction movement is applied to deliver the baby's head, thus avoiding sudden decompression. The forceps are slowly dismantled. Haste will only result in a traumatic rupture of the tentorium cerebelli, with grave consequences.

Fig. 9.19

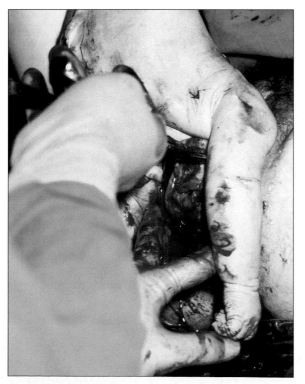

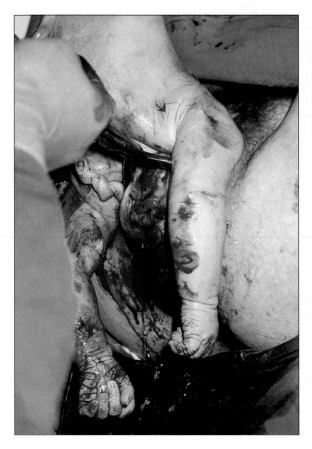

Fig. 9.20

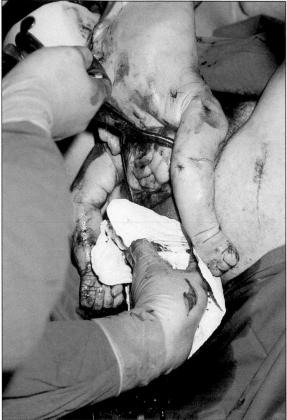

Fig. 9.21

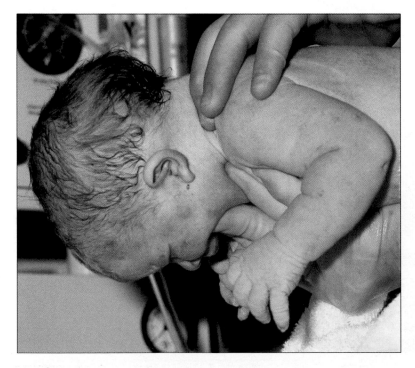

Fig. 9.22 Some obstetricians like to use the Mauriceau–Smellie–Viet technique. The fetal trunk is allowed to ride over the operator's right arm. The operator's right index and middle fingers are placed to exercise pressure against the baby's maxillae, thus maximizing flexion of the baby's head; pressure must not be placed against the baby's lower jaw. The left hand rests on the baby's back, with the left index and ring fingers pulling on his shoulders, and the left middle finger promoting head flexion. Steady and gentle traction allows safe delivery of the infant. However, it must be remembered that such traction is being exerted through the cervical spines and the associated articulations, whereas in the case of a forceps delivery of the after-coming head, traction is applied through the child's entire head.

Chapter TEN

Delivery of Twins

MANAGEMENT OF THE SECOND STAGE OF LABOUR

Twin pregnancy is a high-risk situation – all the physiological changes and complications of pregnancy are more pronounced and, with the exception of using ultrasound scan measurements to determine chorionicity (see **Figs 1.14a–d**) and to monitor fetal growth, the obstetrician is denied the tests of fetal well-being that are available during the management of singleton pregnancies. Twins labour is a high-risk situation for both mother and babies. It carries a greater risk of fetal distress, with the second twin accessible only by external Doppler monitoring, and a higher incidence of operative delivery and maternal bleeding.

During the course of antenatal care, a decision must be made as to the mode of delivery. In general, elective caesarean sections may be performed for cases in which a similar decision would have been taken for a singleton pregnancy – for example, breech presentation of a growth-retarded baby. More specifically, however, elective caesarean section may be performed, for example, when the first twin, presenting by the head, suffers from growth retardation, and when the second twin, of normal size, is presenting by the breech.

The special care baby unit should be informed of a twin labour as soon as the patient is admitted to the delivery suite. During the first stage of labour, an intravenous infusion line is established, and a blood sample is collected for estimation of haemoglobin and for blood grouping, if blood cross-matching facilities are available within a short time; if a rapid service is not available, it is prudent to prepare 2 units of blood. Ten units of oxytocin are diluted in 500 ml of normal saline, and left by the bedside ready for use in the second stage if required.

The course of the second stage of twins labour differs from that of singleton labour, particularly in the organization of personnel. During the second stage, an experienced obstetrician and an assistant, together with the patient's midwife, must be in attendance. An anaesthetist, with an anaesthetic machine, must be present in the labour room, prepared to give general anaesthesia at short notice. Finally, two paediatricians, or at least one and an assistant capable of neonatal resuscitation, must be present in the delivery room, together with two resuscitaires.

In the case of twins delivery illustrated in **Figures 10.1–10.22**, both babies are presenting by the head. The conduct of the second stage of labour for the delivery of the first twin (**Figs 10.1–10.18**) is similar to that of any other singleton birth with cephalic presentation.

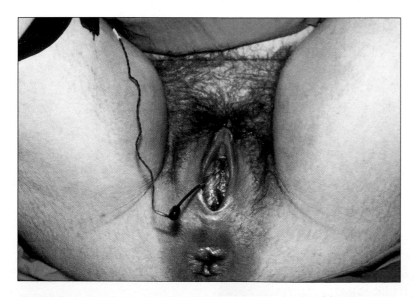

Fig. 10.1 The midwife conducts the delivery as usual. The first twin's heart rate pattern is monitored with a fetal scalp electrode, while the second twin is monitored by ultrasound using a Doppler transducer on the mother's abdomen.

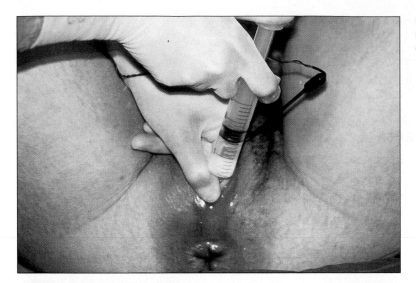

Figs 10.2–10.4 The need for episiotomy necessitates the administration of local anaesthetic.

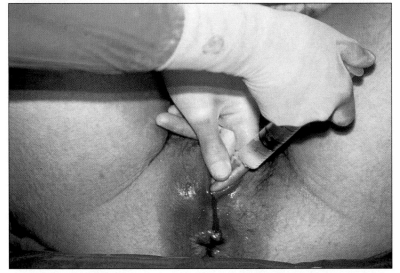

Fig. 10.3

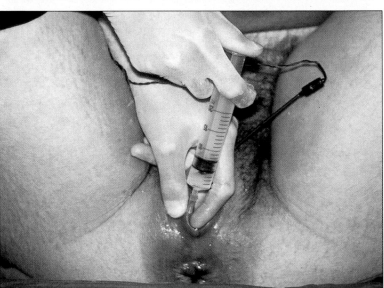

Fig. 10.4

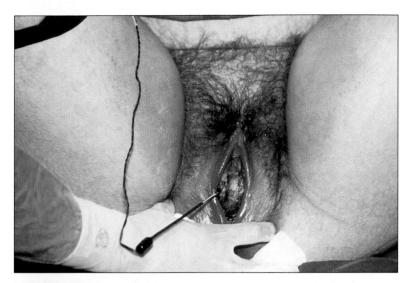

Figs 10.5–10.7 As the vulval tissue becomes more stretched (**Fig. 10.5**), a posterolateral episiotomy is performed with a pair of angled scissors (**Figs 10.6 & 10.7**).

Fig. 10.6

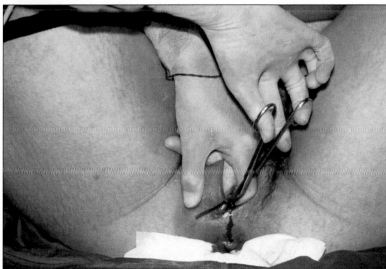

Fig. 10.7

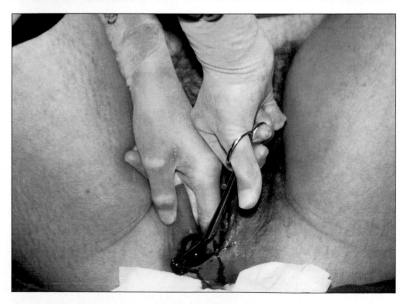

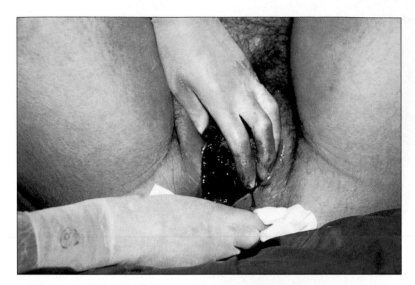

Figs 10.8–10.13 Well-maintained flexion of the head results in the smallest diameter of the fetal skull being presented to the maternal soft tissue. The perineum is well supported with a gauze pad.

Fig. 10.9

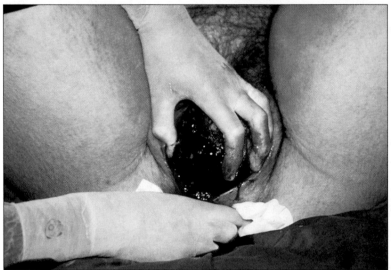

Fig. 10.10

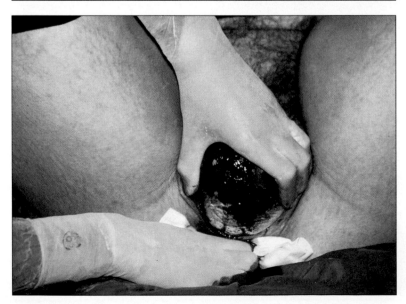

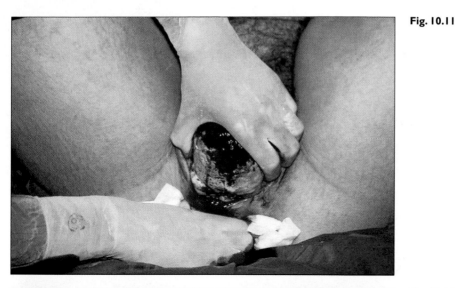

Fig. 10.11

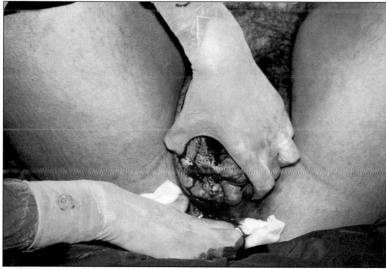

Fig. 10.12

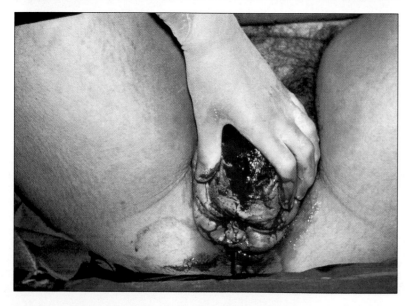

Fig. 10.13

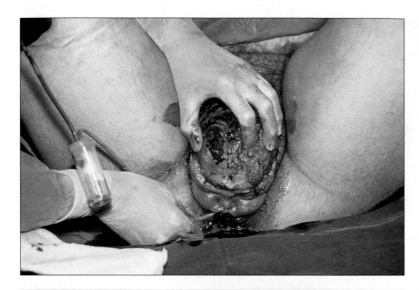

Fig. 10.14 When the head is delivered, the mouth and nostrils are cleared by suction.

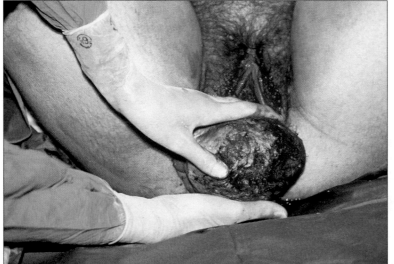

Figs 10.15 & 10.16 After external rotation of the head (**Fig. 10.15**), the anterior shoulder is delivered (**Fig. 10.16**).

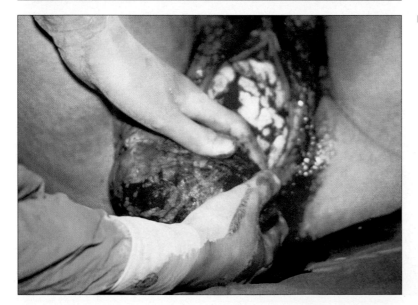

Fig. 10.16

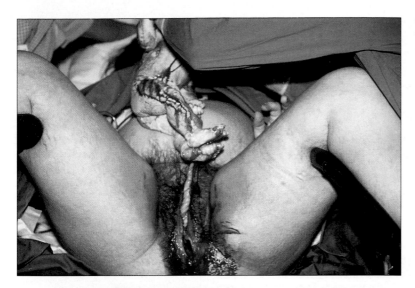

Fig. 10.17 The remainder of the baby then follows. (A note of caution: no oxytocin or syntometrine must be administered at this time, because the second stage is not yet complete – another baby will follow!)

Fig. 10.18 The umbilical cord is clamped, marked and cut.

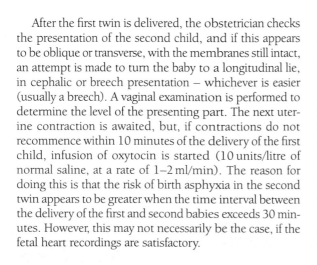

After the first twin is delivered, the obstetrician checks the presentation of the second child, and if this appears to be oblique or transverse, with the membranes still intact, an attempt is made to turn the baby to a longitudinal lie, in cephalic or breech presentation – whichever is easier (usually a breech). A vaginal examination is performed to determine the level of the presenting part. The next uterine contraction is awaited, but, if contractions do not recommence within 10 minutes of the delivery of the first child, infusion of oxytocin is started (10 units/litre of normal saline, at a rate of 1–2 ml/min). The reason for doing this is that the risk of birth asphyxia in the second twin appears to be greater when the time interval between the delivery of the first and second babies exceeds 30 minutes. However, this may not necessarily be the case, if the fetal heart recordings are satisfactory.

If there is evidence of fetal distress or cord prolapse in the second twin, it is possible to deliver the baby by applying a pair of forceps or a ventouse, if the baby is presenting by the head, or by performing breech extraction, as appropriate. In such cases, the author uses Kjelland's forceps for the delivery of the second twin, in order that, should rotation be required, a change of instrument is not necessary. Alternatively, a ventouse can be used, particularly if the head lies 2–3 cm above the ischial spines and there is a need for a quick delivery of the second twin; however, this instrument is appropriate only if the pregnancy is advanced to 35 weeks or more. The sequence of events in such a delivery, from the application of the suction cup to the delivery of the second twin, is depicted in **Figures 10.23–10.33**.

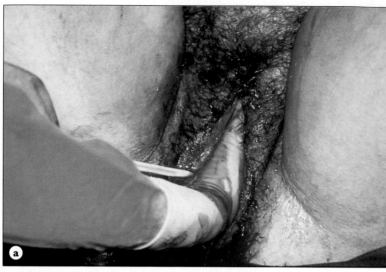

Fig. 10.19a & b When uterine contractions recommence, forcing the presenting part into the pelvis, vaginal examination is repeated, with the intention of artificially rupturing the membranes, if no other problem such as cord presentation is noted, or if the presentation is that of breech. Should the latter be the case, the obstetrician should take over and conduct the delivery, first considering the option of abdominal delivery. Emergency caesarean section may be indicated if it is judged that the course of the second stage may not otherwise be accomplished safely – for example, if the cervix is contracting after the birth of the first twin, and the second twin is presenting by the shoulder or the breech. Artificial rupture of the membranes will allow further descent of the presenting part and the delivery of the second twin.

Figs 10.20–10.22 The head of the second twin is delivered; note the cord of the first twin, which appears in the background.

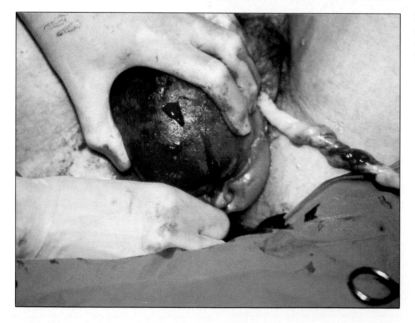

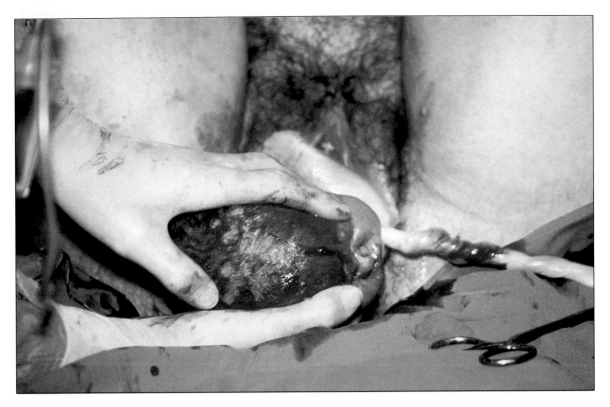

Fig. 10.21 Delivery of the anterior shoulder.

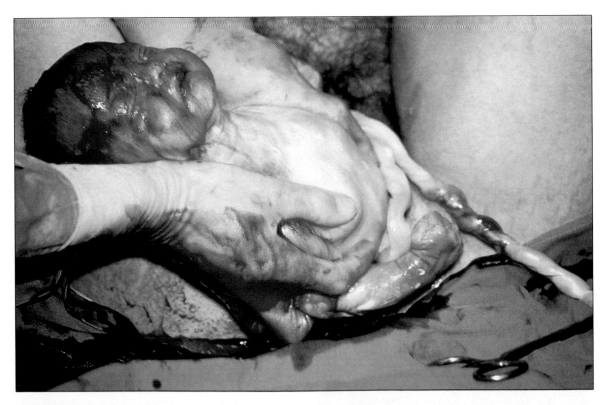

Fig. 10.22 Delivery of the posterior shoulder and the rest of the baby.

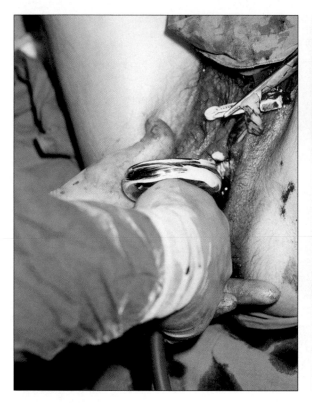

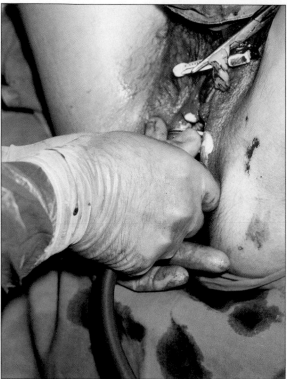

Figs 10.23 & 10.24 Ventouse extraction of the second twin: the suction cup is applied to the baby's head. The operator ensures that no maternal tissue is inadvertently sucked in.

Fig. 10.24

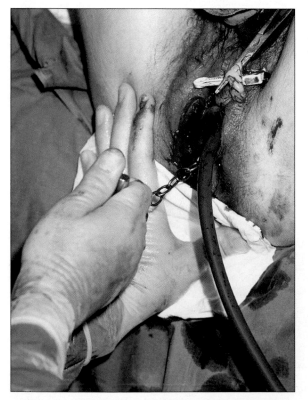

Figs 10.25–10.29 Traction is started in a downwards direction and is progressively curved upwards. The perineum is supported with a gauze pad. Note the sequential change in direction of traction on the chain.

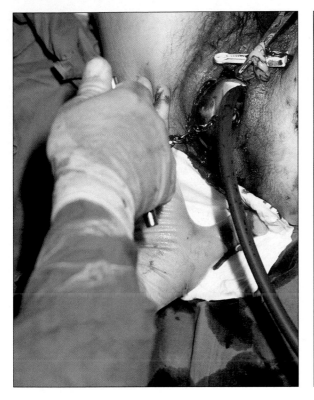

Fig. 10.26

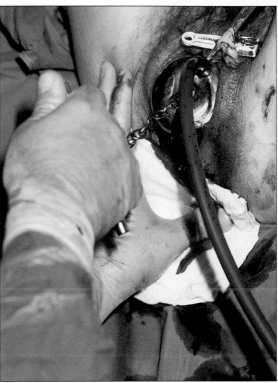

Fig. 10.27

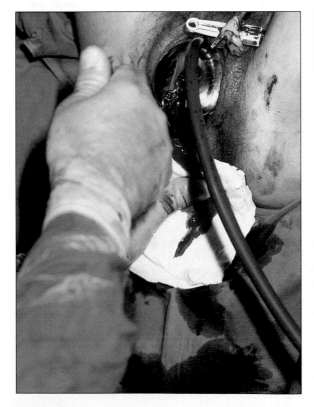

Fig. 10.28

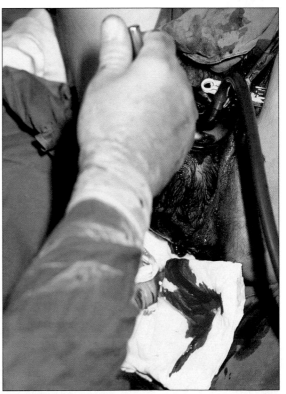

Fig. 10.29

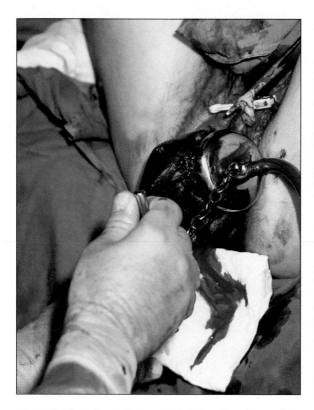

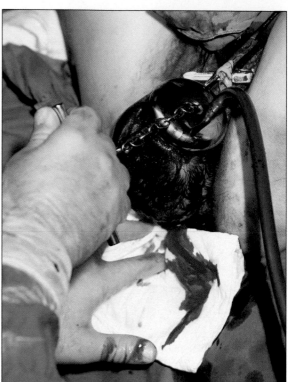

Figs 10.30 & 10.31 Restitution rapidly follows the delivery of the head. The occiput is pointing to 2 o'clock.

Fig. 10.31

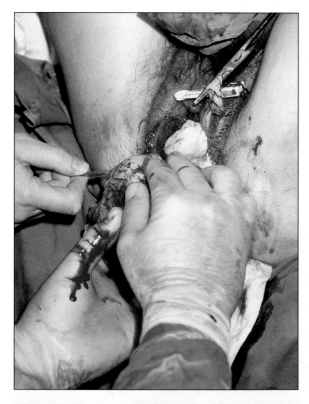

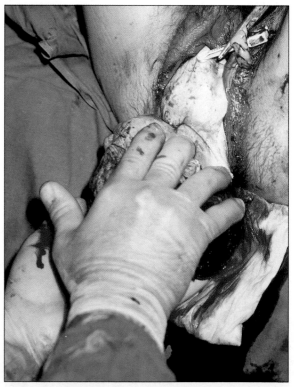

Fig. 10.32 External rotation has taken place and the anterior shoulder appears under the pubic symphysis.

Fig. 10.33 The anterior shoulder is being delivered.

INTERNAL PODALIC VERSION

On occasion, especially when external version is being attempted to correct a transverse lie of the second twin, spontaneous rupture of the membranes may occur, with the resulting prolapse of an arm or leg. If it is a leg that has prolapsed, a straightforward breech extraction is performed, after the obstetrician is satisfied that no contraindications exist. If an arm has prolapsed, it may be necessary to proceed to internal podalic version and breech extraction; in modern obstetrics, this is probably the only situation in which these manoeuvres are regarded as acceptable practice. The induction of general anaesthesia is required, with complete relaxation of the uterus. Caesarean section may be a safer option when delivering the second twin in such circumstances, especially if the obstetrician is not experienced in internal podalic version.

The principle behind successful version is the pulling of the baby's ankle(s) in a direction that promotes the flexion attitude, and therefore facilitates the manoeuvres involved. If this principle is not followed, an arm or a deflexed head may be arrested by the uterine wall.

There are two types of presentation: ventral and dorsal. In ventral presentation, in which the baby is lying with its back to the fundus, all that is required is to reach for the ankle(s) and apply traction to deliver the legs. If the baby's abdomen is facing the uterine fundus, as in dorsal presentation, the ankle is pulled in a composite movement, first to achieve more flexion, and second to turn the baby along its longitudinal axis to convert the presentation into a ventral one, before traction is applied on the baby's ankles for breech extraction. This necessitates careful examination to locate the head and the back. The obstetrician's right hand and forearm, preferably clothed in an elbow-length glove, are introduced into the vagina; the obstetrician searches for a foot inside the uterus, steadying it and its contents with the other hand *per abdomen*. As a foot is grasped and pulled down, the other leg follows (**Fig. 10.34**). Both legs are then grasped by the ankles and steadily pulled until the buttocks are delivered. The obstetrician grasps the fetus gently but firmly by the buttocks, with the palms of his hands. Traction is applied until the lower angle of the shoulder blades (scapulae) is seen, maintaining the baby's back upwards all the time. The arms are searched for in the vagina and are delivered in the same way as described in breech presentation. If the arms are extended, they are delivered by Lövset's manoeuvre.

The baby is then allowed to hang by the body, resulting in further descent of the head into the lower part of the pelvis. The delivery of the after-coming head is described on pp. 119–122.

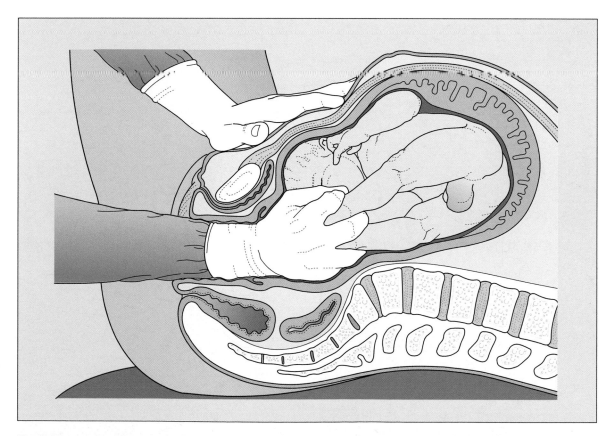

Fig. 10.34 Internal podalic version: the operator introduces a hand into the uterine cavity and attempts to grasp a foot or both feet. To facilitate the procedure, the other hand is used to push the head, *per abdomen*, in the other direction.

Caesarean Section

The operation of caesarean section is a technique whereby the course of childbirth is interrupted, and delivery via the natural passages is rejected in favour of the abdominal route. Over the past 50 years this procedure, which used to be reserved for women whose lives were already in jeopardy because of pregnancy and labour, has acquired a long list of indications. These can be summarized to encompass two main categories: maternal and fetal. The former include pelvic contracture attributable to bony or soft-tissue factors, uterine muscle 'failure' or inertia, and poor metabolic performance that makes labour a hazardous experience, for example poorly controlled diabetes mellitus or severe pre-eclampsia. Fetal indications for caesarean section mainly concern the presence of hypoxia and acidosis, but also include those cases in which mechanical difficulties are anticipated for the baby during its passage through the birth canal: for example, a large or a very small baby, abnormal presentation, prolapse of the umbilical cord or fetal abnormalities. An indication for caesarean section can also result from factors that affect both mother and child, such as placenta praevia.

The number of caesarean sections has increased steeply over the past 30 years and has closely reflected an identical increase in the rate of induction of labour. The operation has sometimes been so frequently deemed to be indicated that critics have described it as the panacea of obstetric practice. Factors promoting its increase include the increasing safety of the procedure, with the introduction of better anaesthesia, blood transfusion and more effective antibiotics. The wide recourse to caesarean section has also been prompted by an increase in the number of litigations brought against obstetricians, for alleged negligence.

Epidemiological evidence for the association of mental and physical handicap with genetic and environmental factors, particularly prenatal events, has emerged only recently. The studies concerned have also demonstrated that the majority of cases of childhood handicap, physical and mental, are not associated with adverse intrapartum factors.

LOWER SEGMENT CAESAREAN SECTION

Lower segment caesarean section is the procedure performed most commonly, the classical *midline upper segment* caesarean being reserved for the rare occasion of transverse lie in labour when the liquor amnii has drained away, after spontaneous rupture of the membranes. The reason for preferring the lower segment technique is that it is associated with a lower incidence of dehiscence of the uterine scar in subsequent pregnancy.

Another type of lower segment operation is the *longitudinal lower segment* incision of De Lee (see pp. 146-153). This is a very useful alternative to lower segment or classical caesarean section in the delivery of small babies, particularly those presenting by the breech when the lower segment is still thick. The incidence of dehiscence of the scar in De Lee's operation is reported to be as low as that of the transverse lower segment operation.

Anaesthesia. The types of anaesthesia used for caesarean section include general and conduction anaesthesia, which may be an epidural, spinal or even a local infiltration, although the last is rarely used in present-day practice.

Position. A cushion wedge is fitted under the right loin, to direct the weight of the gravid uterus away from the inferior vena cava and thus avoid supine hypotension syndrome.

Preparation. The bladder is emptied by catheterization. The skin of the anterior abdominal wall is cleaned with antiseptic solution, such as chlorhexidine in spirit, and the patient is draped.

Technique

Figures 11.1–11.15 illustrate a lower segment caesarean section up to the stage of delivery. When the uterus has retracted after the delivery of the child, the placenta is delivered by controlled cord traction, and the empty state of the uterus is confirmed by digital examination. The operator's index finger is passed through the cervical canal from above, to ensure that it is open. The Doyen retractor is re-introduced, and Green-Armytage forceps are applied to the angles of the uterine incision and to any major bleeding vessel at the edge of the uterine wound.

The wound is closed in two layers with No. 0 Vicryl suture. The first layer of continuous suturing excludes the decidua and involves about two-thirds of the thickness of the edge of the uterine wound (**Figs 11.16–11.18**). The second continuous suture includes the superficial layer (the remaining one-third) of the uterine muscles, and buries the first suture line (**Figs 11.19–11.25**).

When haemostasis is satisfactory, the ovaries are examined to ensure that no neoplastic cysts are present; it is rather embarrassing if an ovarian cyst undergoes torsion during the puerperium after caesarean section. The incised edges of the uterovesical folds of the peritoneum are

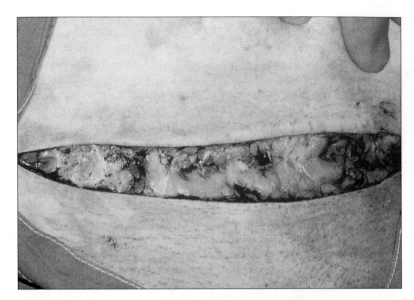

Fig. 11.1 Lower section caesarean section: the abdomen is opened through a skin incision performed with a scalpel (size 4) transversely, 4 cm above the symphysis pubis. The curved incision, 18–20 cm in length, is made along the lower abdominal crease, its concavity directed cephalad.

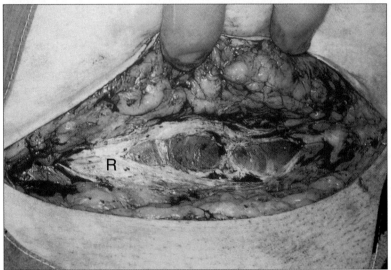

Fig. 11.2 The subcutaneous fat is incised down to the anterior rectus sheath (R), which is then incised with a scalpel, on either side of the midline.

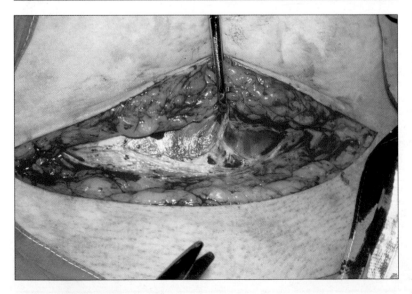

Figs 11.3 & 11.4 This opening is enlarged bilaterally, and the recti are separated from the overlying rectus sheath, using curved scissors. The bladder (B) is visible (**Fig. 11.4**).

Fig. 11.4

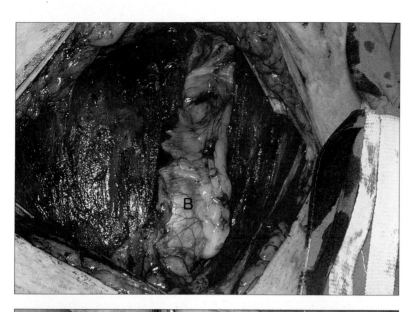

Figs 11.5 & 11.6 The peritoneum is then opened longitudinally in the midline, by about 1–2 cm, and the incision is enlarged transversely to avoid the dome of the bladder. (Adhesions of the uterovesical peritoneal reflection are clearly visible here, and are due to a previous caesarean section.)

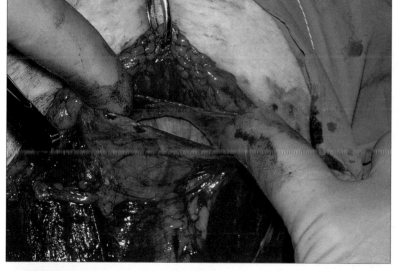

Fig. 11.6

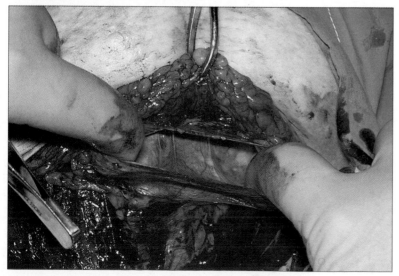

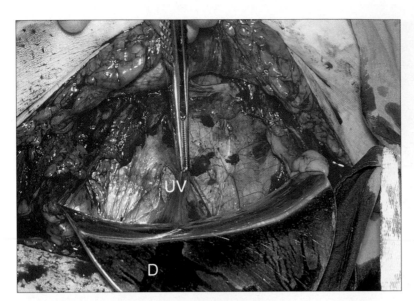

Figs 11.7 & 11.8a & b A Doyen retractor (D) is inserted to expose the uterovesical fold (UV) of the peritoneum. An abdominal pack is inserted on each side of the uterus, to limit the escape of liquor and vernix into the peritoneal cavity. The uterovesical peritoneum is lifted with dissecting forceps and incised with scissors, to both the left and the right. The bladder is then pushed downwards and held under the Doyen retractor. The peritoneum is, in this case, rather adherent to the underlying uterine muscle tissue, as a result of a previous caesarean section.

Fig. 11.8a

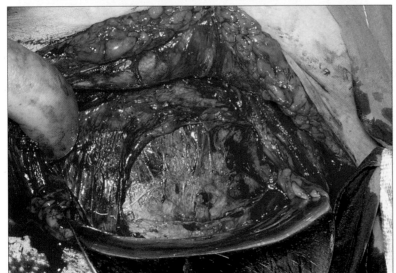

Fig. 11.8b

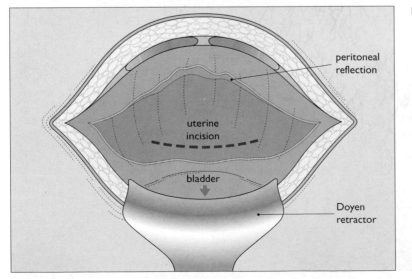

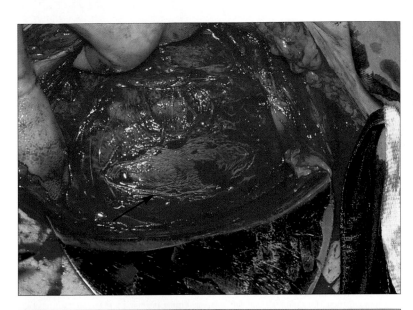

Fig. 11.9 A shallow incision is then made with a scalpel, across the lower uterine segment and curving slightly upwards at each end (arrow). This incision is deepened until the uterine cavity is entered.

The incision is then extended, by tearing with the two index fingers along the line of the shallow incision.

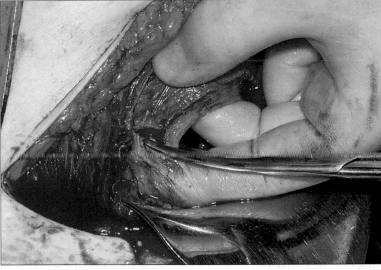

Figs 11.10 & 11.11 An alternative technique, and one followed by the author, is to hold a slightly opened pair of curved scissors against the end of the uterine incision and, by pushing these against the uterine muscle, tearing and splitting (but not cutting) the muscle fibres in a slightly upwardly curving line. Appropriate precautions must be taken to avoid injury to the baby. This technique is particularly useful when caesarean section is being performed after a prolonged labour, for example towards the end of the first stage of labour, or if the operation is performed in the second stage. In these instances the lower segment is very thin, and the practice of tearing the uterine muscle with two fingers (as in **Fig. 11.9**) may cause the uterine wound to extend into the broad ligament, or may even result in the tear of the lower segment extending into the vagina.

Fig. 11.11

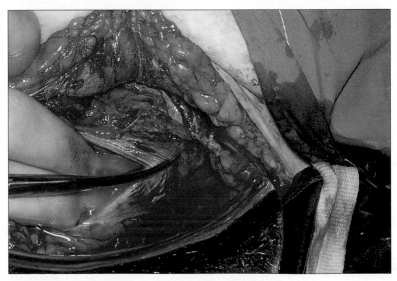

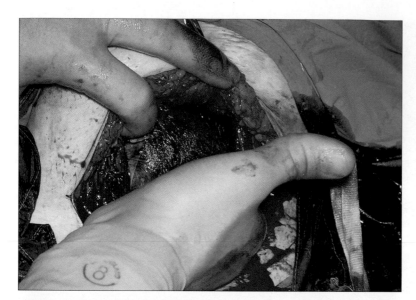

Figs 11.12 & 11.13 The surgeon's right hand is inserted under the fetal head, which is levered out through the uterine wound. At this point, the Doyen retractor is removed. The baby's nostrils and mouth are cleared by suction as soon as the head is delivered. The rest of the baby is delivered by the application of traction on the baby's head, as the assistant applies pressure on the uterine fundus.

The cord is clamped and cut between two artery forceps, and the baby passed to the attending paediatrician.

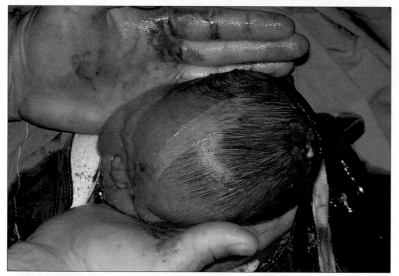

Fig. 11.13

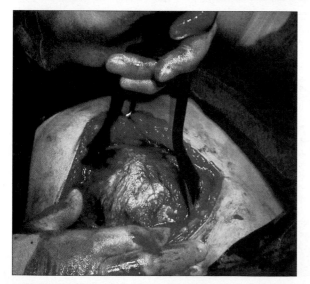

Fig. 11.14 The alternative technique, particularly in the case of a high head, is to deliver the baby's head via the application of forceps.

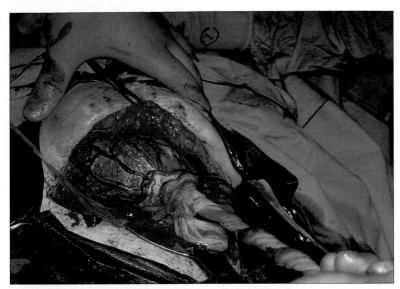

Fig. 11.15 At the moment of delivery of the head, the anaesthetist gives 10 units of oxytocin intravenously, or one ampoule of syntometrine intramuscularly.

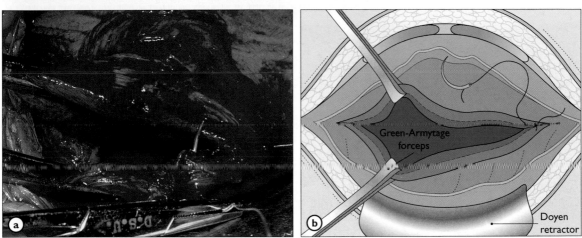

Figs 11.16a & b & 11.17a & b Wound closure: suturing starts at the left angle (**Fig. 11.16**) and is continued towards the right angle (**Fig. 11.17**).

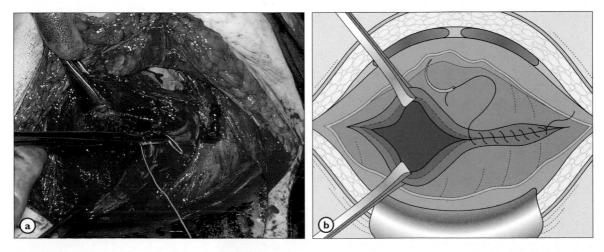

Fig. 11.17

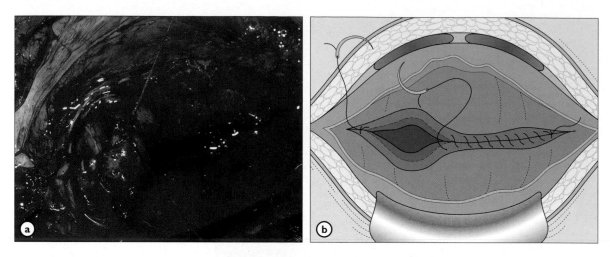

Fig. 11.18a & b Half-way through suturing, however, the author secures the right angle with a separate stitch (full-length suture), making certain that apposition and haemostasis are well accomplished. The first suture is continued and tied at the right corner of the uterine wound.

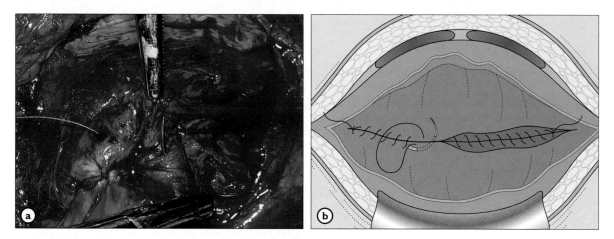

Fig. 11.19a & b The second layer is sutured from the right angle to the left, in a continuous fashion. The edges of the uterovesical peritoneal fold are sutured in the following step

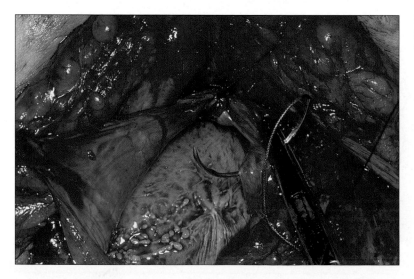

Figs 11.20 & 11.21 The parietal peritoneum is closed with No. 2/0 Vicryl suture.

Fig. 11.21

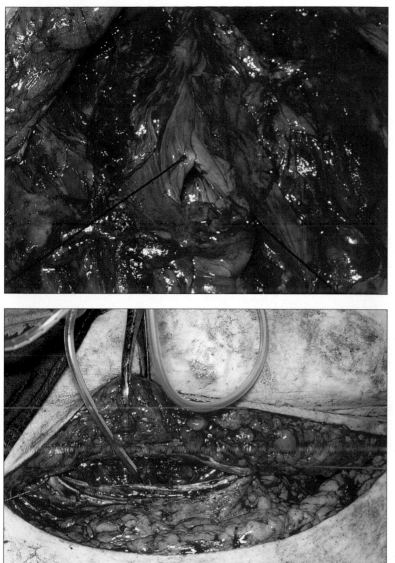

Fig. 11.22 The rectus sheath is closed with No. 0 Vicryl. Other sutures may be used, for example No. 0 Nylon sutures.

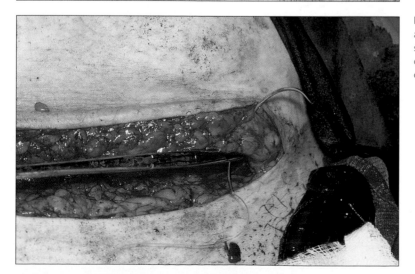

Fig. 11.23 The subcutaneous fat is approximated with No. 00 plain cat-gut suture, in order to support the skin edges; otherwise, the scar will sink below the level of the skin.

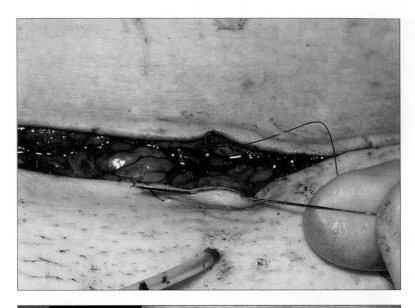

Figs 11.24 & 11.25 Clips, staples and interrupted nylon sutures are all in use to close the skin, but a subcuticular proline suture gives an excellent result.

Fig. 11.25

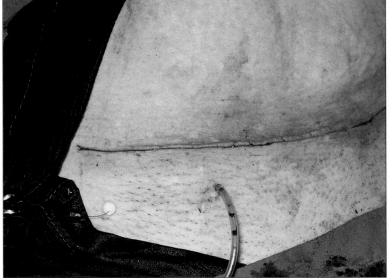

repaired with a continuous suture, using No. 2/0 Vicryl. The blood clots and liquor are removed from the peritoneal cavity. The parietal peritoneum is closed with No. 2/0 Vicryl in a continuous suture.

A Redivac drain is usually left under the sheath for 24–48 hours until it stops draining. In the author's experience, rectus sheath haematomas occur only rarely when this technique is used.

ABDOMINAL DELIVERY OF THE SMALL BABY

If the lower segment has not yet formed, a lower segment caesarean section may be technically difficult to perform, particularly when dealing with, for example, the preterm infant presenting by the breech at 26–32 weeks' gestation, with severe pre-eclampsia. If the uterus is opened in the usual way, through a transverse incision of the lower segment, the incision is usually small and the upper edge of the wound too thick – a combination that may limit access, hinder manipulation and delivery and necessitate strong traction on the baby. It is in circumstances such as these that De Lee's vertical lower segment incision is preferable.

VERTICAL LOWER SEGMENT CAESAREAN SECTION (DE LEE'S OPERATION)
(Figs 11.26–11.43)

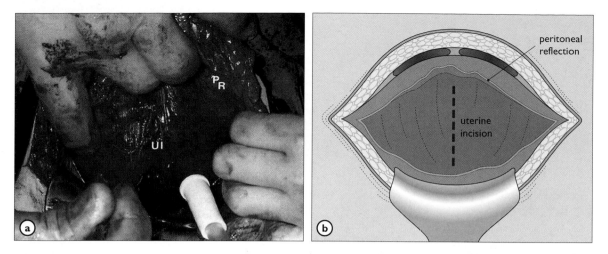

Fig. 11.26a & b De Lee's operation: after the bladder is reflected from the lower part of the uterus, the uterus is incised longitudinally in the midline with a scalpel.

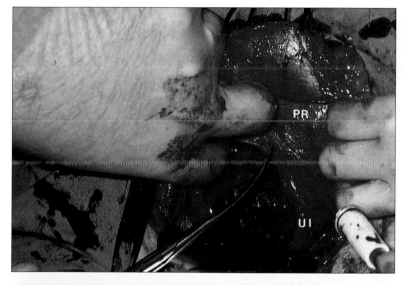

Figs 11.27 & 11.28 The length of the incision is about 10 cm from the upper limit of the cervix, assessed by palpation, to the peritoneal reflection (PR) on the uterus. UI = uterine incision.

When the cavity is entered, the incision is completed throughout the thickness of the uterine wall as the operator tears the muscle fibres with a pair of curved scissors, guiding them with his fingers to avoid injury to the baby.

Fig. 11.28

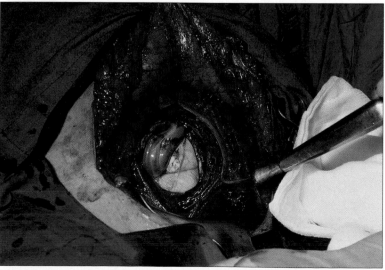

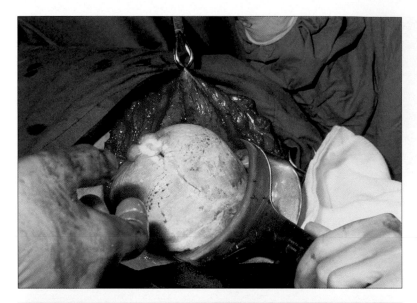

Fig. 11.29 The operator's hand is inserted under the presenting part, breech in this case, which is levered outside the uterine wound. At this stage the Doyen retractor is removed.

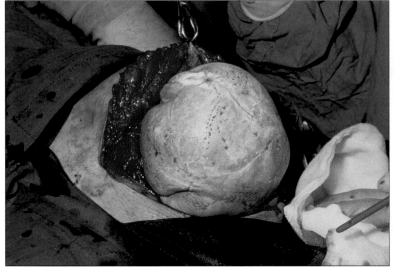

Figs 11.30–11.32 Fundal pressure is gently applied by the assistant, to deliver the breech slowly.

Fig. 11.31

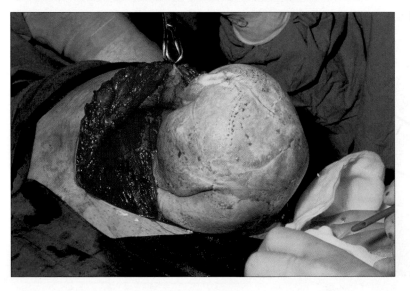

Fig. 11.32

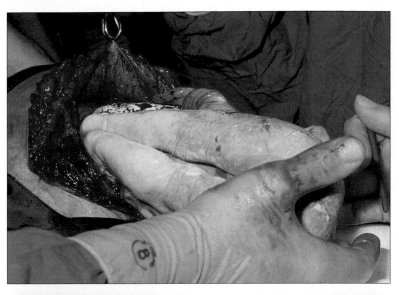

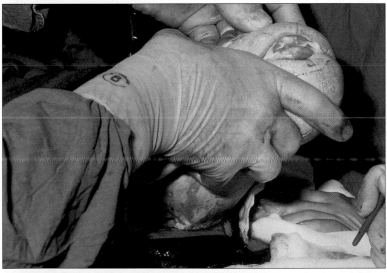

Fig. 11.33 As delivery is accomplished up to the level of the scapulae, the arms are helped out of the uterine wound.

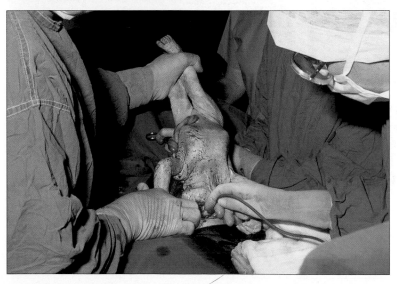

Fig. 11.34 The after-coming head is now in the lower uterine segment. The baby is held up by the ankles and swung towards the maternal chest, exposing the mouth and nostrils for clearance by suction. Well-controlled delivery of the after-coming head is as important during caesarean section for breech presentation as during vaginal delivery, because sudden compression–decompression may result in tentorial tears, particularly in these small babies.

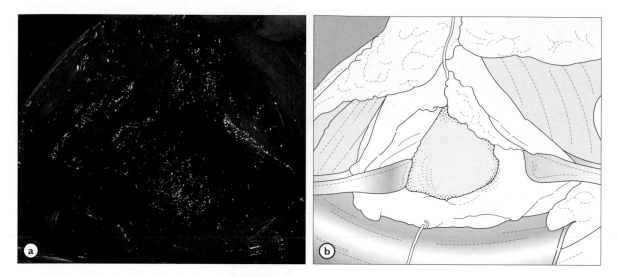

Fig. 11.35a & b The uterus immediately after delivery. When the inferior corner of the incision is secured, Green-Armytage forceps are applied to each side of the uterine wound.

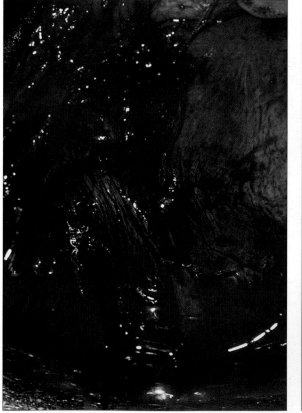

Fig. 11.36 The first layer of suturing of the uterine wall starts at the superior angle; continuous suturing with No. 0 Vicryl completes the first layer, which incorporates the inner two-thirds of the wall thickness, but avoids the decidua.

Figs 11.37 & 11.38 The second layer of suturing starts at the inferior angle, and approximates the outer one-third of each side of the uterine wall, using continuous No. 0 Vicryl.

Blood and vernix are now removed from the wound. Both ovaries are inspected at this stage, to ensure the absence of pathology.

Fig. 11.38

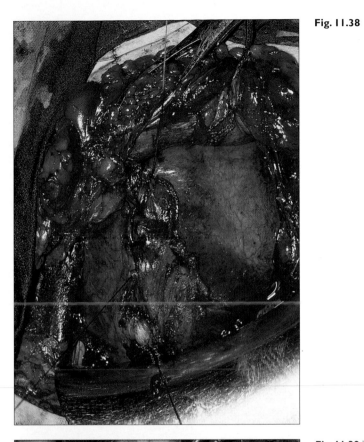

Fig. 11.39 The uterovesical peritoneal fold is refashioned using continuous Vicryl sutures, after haemostasis has been confirmed to be satisfactory. It is perhaps most advantageous to avoid a watertight layer, and to leave a window in the peritoneum of the uterovesical fold. Thus, if a haematoma forms, it can drain into the peritoneal cavity; otherwise, if it remains under the peritoneum, it may cause ileus.

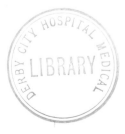

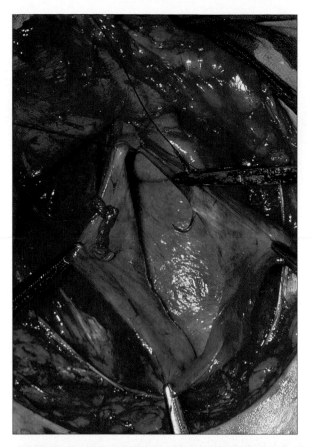

Fig. 11.40 The author closes the parietal peritoneum by everting its edges, a procedure that may help to reduce the formation of adhesions, as it prevents a situation in which a long line of damaged peritoneal edges heals within the peritoneal cavity.

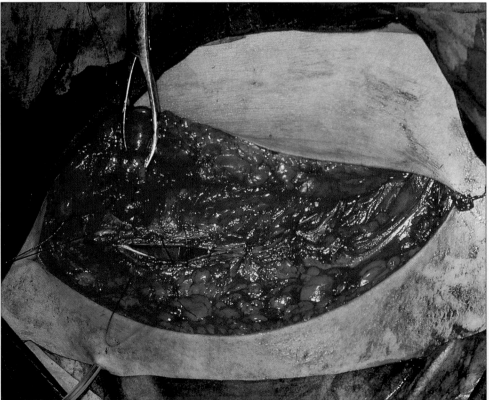

Fig. 11.41 The rectus sheath is sutured with No. 0 Vicryl sutures, after the introduction of a Redivac drain.

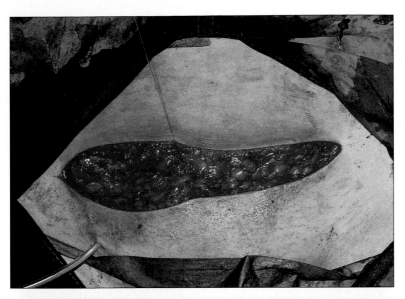

Fig. 11.42 The subcutaneous fat layer is approximated with plain cat-gut sutures. These help to obliterate a dead space and reduce tension on the skin sutures.

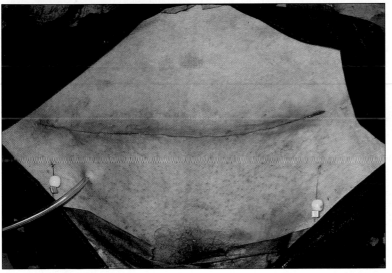

Fig. 11.43 The skin is sutured with subcuticular proline. Note that the ends of the suture are left loose; this allows for postsurgical swelling, thus reducing tension on the skin edges.

'EN CAULE' CAESAREAN SECTION FOR DELIVERY OF THE VERY LOW BIRTHWEIGHT BABY

Although the obstetric problems surrounding the delivery of very low birthweight infants remain unsolved, there have been trends towards a more interventionalist obstetric approach, with caesarean section being an increasingly favoured option. Even though significantly better survival rates have been claimed for infants of less than 1500 g delivered by caesarean section, delivery trauma remains an important obstetric factor.

Two major objectives in the management of preterm delivery are the avoidance of asphyxia and of trauma. The tissues of the preterm baby are easily damaged: excessive moulding of the soft cranium may result in cerebral haemorrhage, and venous engorgement resulting from hypoxia and hypercarbia makes the tentorium more susceptible to injury. The incidence of periventricular haemorrhage among infants weighing less than 1500 g is about 8%.

The earliest gestational age at which caesarean section is performed for fetal indications is decreasing, and the threshold has now retreated to 28 weeks or less. It is nevertheless widely appreciated that caesarean section does not provide the complete solution. At operation there may be difficulties in delivering the head because of a poorly formed lower segment and the need to extend the incision in 7% of operations. These difficulties are compounded by pre-existing malpresentation. Among babies delivered by caesarean section, those presenting by the breech are twice as likely to be depressed at birth as are their cephalic counterparts, and, in the very premature infant, entrapment of the after-coming head is a serious complication, even with the classical incision.

In the author's experience, the main reason why an infant was difficult to extract has seemed to be that, once the membranes were ruptured, the uterus tended to contract and would mould about the fetus, in a manner reminiscent of the so-called 'hug-me-tight' uterus described by earlier writers; unless the surgeon then acted quickly, entrapment problems might occur, causing a further delay in delivery. This latter problem is found most commonly with the after-coming head of the breech baby, the head being larger than the thorax: Usher and McLean (see Further Reading), for instance, showed that the mean circumference of the head at 31 weeks is 28.7 cm, which is 4.7 cm more than the circumference of the thorax.

If the bag of membranes could be allowed to remain intact after the uterine incision had been made, it might be quite easy to deliver the entire gestation sac (including the placenta if necessary) in one piece, thus totally eliminating trauma. Under these circumstances, differences of fetal presentation would also become inconsequential. Because of the anatomy of placentation in the human, the fetal circulation is separate from that of the mother, so that, provided the correct plane of cleavage is identified, there should be no fetal bleeding when the placenta is separated. The 'en caule' technique offers just such a procedure.

Technique

Figures 11.44–11.55 illustrate the technique of 'en caule' caesarean section.

If the placenta is anteriorly placed, it is initially encountered when the uterus is excised. The technique remains essentially the same as above: manual separation of the placenta in the plane of the choriodecidual space, followed by digital separation of the membranes and removal of the intact sac. On no account should the fetal surface of the placenta be incised or otherwise injured, as this may cause fetal bleeding.

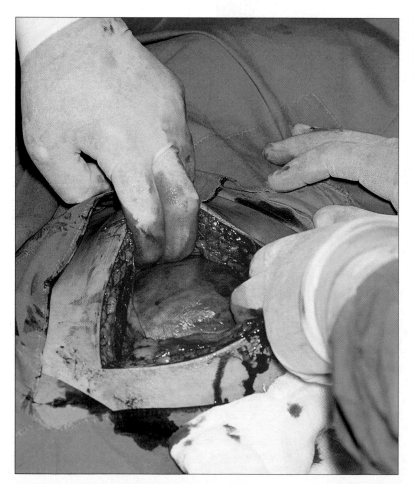

Fig. 11.44 'En caule' caesarean section: with the anaesthetized patient in the lateral tilt position, a midline suprapubic incision is made, to ensure that the tissues of the abdominal wall do not hinder subsequent manoeuvres.

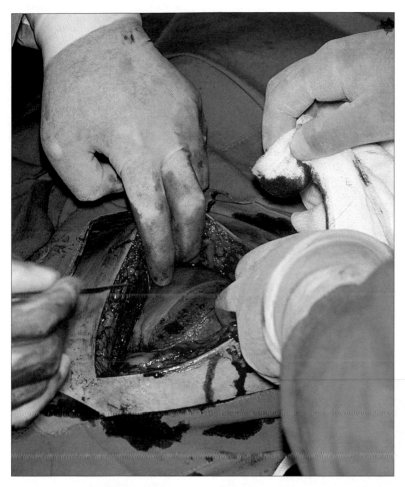

Fig. 11.45 The uterine surface is inspected and, as is usually the case at gestational ages of less than 32 weeks when the mother is not in labour, the lower segment is found to be unformed and very thick.

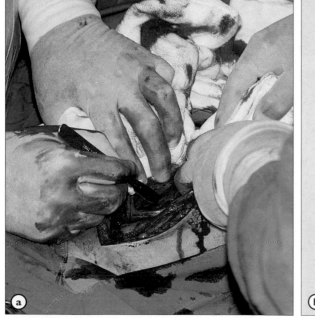

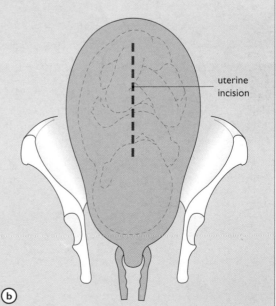

Fig. 11.46a & b A generous midline incision is made in the uterus as far as the fetal membranes.

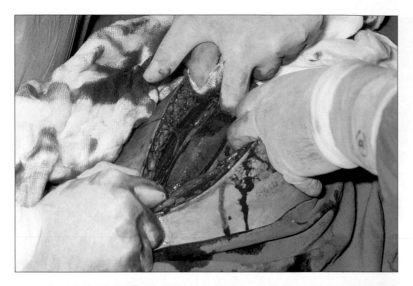

Fig. 11.47 When the membranes are clearly visible, the incision is gently extended using blunt-pointed scissors, and finally digitally stretched to its fullest extent.

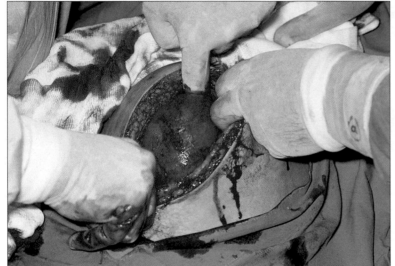

Fig. 11.48 The obstetrician's fingers are inserted into the space between the decidua and the membranes and, with a fish-tailing motion, the amniotic sac is freed as far as possible.

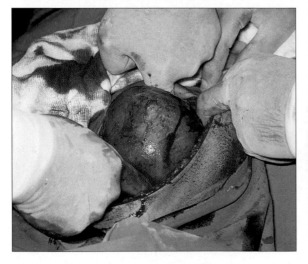

Fig. 11.49 This results in the amniotic sac bulging out of the wound, with the fetus contained within it.

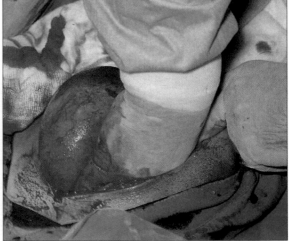

Figs 11.50–11.52 The sac can then be lifted out in an intact state. Note the placental surface.

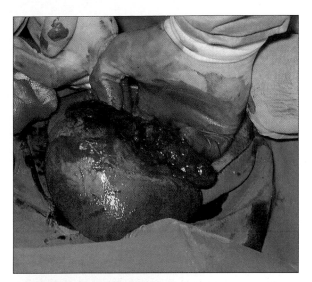

Fig. 11.51

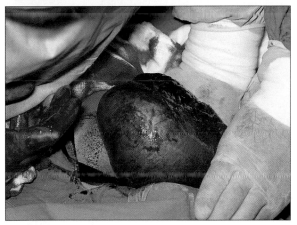

Fig. 11.52

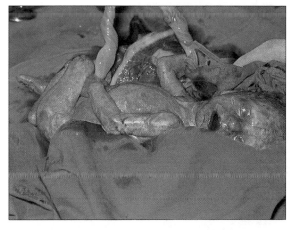

Fig. 11.53 The sac is carefully opened and the baby is taken by the attending paediatrician.

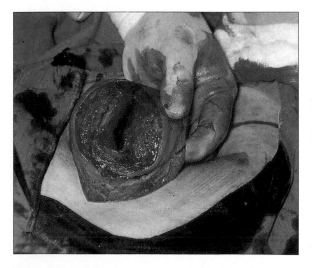

Fig. 11.54 The uterus immediately after delivery.

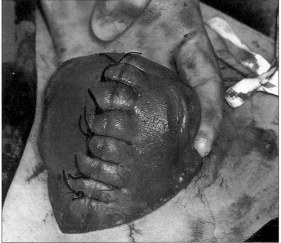

Fig. 11.55 Closure of the uterus, using No. 1 silk in a monolayer.

If the patient is in labour and the membranes are still intact, their integrity should always be preserved.

Inspection of the lower segment may show that a lower segment has in fact formed and that a lower segment caesarean section is a reasonable option. Under these circumstances, the lower segment incision is made in the usual way, without rupturing the membranes. The transverse incision is stretched digitally to its full lateral extent. The membranes are then carefully separated digitally from the lower margin of the incision, in such a way that a hand can then be inserted below the membranes onto the lower part of the posterior wall of the uterus. Intrinsic uterine tone, with a little fundal pressure, causes the membranes to bulge out from the lower segment enclosing the fetus. After the fetus has been 'exteriorized' in this way, the membranes are ruptured. The placenta in this situation seldom presents an obstacle, and the removal of the entire gestation sac in the case of the lower segment operation is not usually necessary.

If the classical uterine incision is used, the standard, layered closure technique using chromic cat-gut, which dates from the latter part of the nineteenth century, has several disadvantages, including foreign-body reaction and resulting poor scar integrity. As a method of closure, the author uses the full thickness of the myometrium, using No. 1 silk in a monolayer of interrupted sutures. This method of closure is quick and easy. Among Potter & Johnston's 1954 series of 1521 cases, rupture of the uteri did not occur, and they claimed that histological examination of excised uterine scars showed healing to be superior to that of incisions sutured by layered cat-gut. Certainly the method is very quick, easy and neat, and seems to offer an improvement on others.

Discussion

Very low birthweight infants account for fewer than 1% of all births and, of these, about 70% occur in women in spontaneous labour, 30% of whom will have ruptured membranes at the time of their admission to hospital. Elective delivery of very low birthweight infants is thus an uncommon event, most frequently occasioned by fulminating pre-eclampsia, and more rarely following progressive antepartum haemorrhage or antenatal fetal distress with a 'small for dates' infant.

The application of the technique of 'en caule' caesarean section is clearly limited to those patients with intact membranes; in view of this, it would seem prudent to avoid deliberately rupturing the membranes of women who are carrying very low birthweight infants. For instance, should a woman in spontaneous preterm labour at less than 32 weeks develop strong evidence of fetal asphyxia indicating caesarean section, it would be inadvisable to rupture the membranes in order to observe the colour of the liquor or for purposes of fetal scalp blood sampling: such action might well render the caesarean section much more difficult, and expose the infant to the dangers of mechanical trauma that, added to asphyxia, portend a grim prognosis. The author strongly advocates the preservation of the membranes whenever possible, even at the expense of having to rely solely on the fetal heart rate pattern for the diagnosis of fetal asphyxia; when the consequences of error are certain to be disastrous, it is hardly possible to be too careful.

The benefits of this type of operative procedure are theoretical rather than proven. Indeed, the place of even conventional caesarean section has not been clearly established in dealing with very low birthweight infants. This is not surprising, because of the heterogeneous nature of the very low birthweight population, not to mention the confounding effects of maternal disease, maternal medication and the differing levels of fetal aerobiosis that are likely to be encountered when delivery is necessary at such an early gestational age. However, at the very least, the 'en caule' caesarean section virtually guarantees the delivery of an infant free from physical trauma and therefore deserves serious consideration if the chances of survival of an intact fetus are to be maximized.

Finally, it is important to remember that the fetal anomaly rate is increased in compromised infants at this gestational age: about 8% for breech infants of 32 weeks. It thus behoves the obstetrician to exclude such anomalies whenever possible before surgery. However, as many of them are not readily amenable to diagnosis, liberal use of caesarean section will, from time to time, result in seriously abnormal or non-viable babies.

Note: The author of this atlas has used the 'en caule' caesarean section technique on numerous occasions, through the lower segment incision, for babies up to 38 weeks' gestation. It has been particularly useful in delivering growth-retarded babies in breech presentation, and in cases of placenta praevia. In the latter instances, bleeding has been remarkably minimal.

Further Reading

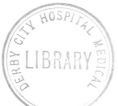

K. Boddy, I.J.T. Parboosingh, W.C. Shepherd, *A Schematic Approach to Prenatal Care* (Edinburgh University, Edinburgh).

W.E. Brenner, R.D. Bruce, C.H. Hendrick, 'The characteristics and perils of breech presentation', *Am J Obstet Gynecol*, **118** (1974), 700–712.

J.A. Chalmers, *The Ventouse, The Obstetric Vacuum* (Lloyd-Luke Medical Books, 1971).

G. Chamberlain, E. Phillips, B. Howlett, K. Masters, 'British Birth', *Obstetric Care* (William Heinemann, London, 1978), vol. 2, p.197.

S.M. Donn, R.G. Faix, 'Long term prognosis for the infant with severe birth trauma', *Clin Perinatol*, **10** (1983), 507–520.

N.M. Duignan, J.W.W. Studd, A.D Hughes, 'Characteristics of normal labour in different racial groups', *Br J Obstet Gynaecol*, **82** (1975), 593–603.

J.S. Fairbairn, *A Textbook for Midwives*, 5th edn (Humphrey Milford, Oxford University Press, Oxford, 1930).

E.A Friedman, *Labor, Clinical Evaluation and Management* (Meredith Corporation, New York, 1967).

K.H. Nicolaides, P.W. Soothill, 'Cordocentesis', *Progress in Obstetrics and Gynaecology*, ed. J.W. Studd (Churchill Livingstone, London, 1989), vol. 7, pp.123–143.

K. O'Driscoll, D. Meagher, *The Active Management of Labour* (Saunders, London, 1980).

E. Parry Jones, *Kjelland's Forceps* (Butterworth & Co. Ltd, London, 1952).

M. Potter, D.C. Johnston, 'Uterine closure in caesarean section', *Am J Obstet Gynecol*, **67** (1954), 760–767.

E. Saling, *Fetal and Neonatal Hypoxia in Relation to Clinical Obstetric Practice* (Edward Arnold, London, 1968).

S.A. Steel, M. Pearce, 'Delivery of the very low birthweight baby', *Br J Hosp Med*, **36** (1986), 328–341.

K.S. Stewart, 'The Second Stage', *Progress in Obstetrics and Gynaecology*, ed. J.W. Studd (Churchill Livingstone, London, 1984) vol. 4, pp.197–216.

J. Studd, *The Management of Labour* (Blackwell Scientific Publications, London, 1985).

R. Usher, F. McLean, 'Intra-uterine growth of live-born Caucasian infants at sea-level; standards obtained from measurements in seven dimensions of infants born between 25 and 44 weeks' gestation', *J Paediatr.*, **74** (1969), 901–910.

M. Westgren, I. Ingemarsson, H. Ahlstrom, M. Lindroth, N.W. Svenningson, 'Delivery and longterm outcome of very low birthweight infants', *Acta Obstet Gynecol Scand*, **61** (1982), 25–30.

J.S. Wigglesworth, 'Intrapartum and early neonatal death: the interaction of asphyxia and trauma in perinatal pathology', *Major Problems in Pathology*, ed. J.S. Wigglesworth (W.B. Saunders, London, 1984), vol. 15, pp.93–112.

Williams Obstetrics, eds. L.M. Hellman, J.A. Pritchard, 14th edn (Meredith Corporation, New York, 1971).

Williams Obstetrics, eds. F.G. Cunningham, P.C. McDonald, N.F. Gant, K.J. Leveno, L.C. Gilstrap, G.D.V. Hankins, S.L Clark. 20th edn (Prentice Hall International Inc., New York, 1997).

V.Y.H. Yu, B. Bajuk, D. Cutting, A.A. Orgill, J. Astbury, 'Effect of mode of delivery on outcome of very low birthweight infants', *Br J Obstet Gynaecol*, **91** (1984), 633–639.

Index